We hear ourselves best
in the quiet

Light a candle and breathe in

Hold this book close to your heart and ask it a question

Open where you feel guided.
There's a message for you there.

Author, writer, medicine woman, mother, grandmother,
a protector of those she loves,
she is an advocate for those without a voice.
She is here to raise the vibration of the feminine
through words, ritual and plant medicine!

INTRODUCTION
BY LYNETTE ALLEN

It was New Year's eve 2022 and as the world was getting ready for celebrations, parties, get-togethers, I was sat on my own, on my porch on the edge of a Balinese jungle thinking...'This is the year I turn fifty...half a century!'.

That felt crazy and amazing and also very, very special. 'I actually lived that long!', I thought to myself. I finally felt like I might have grown up...formally, you know? But then again, I said that about forty!

I did feel like an honouring was needed. Something. I took that intention into meditation that evening, I sat on the deck and closed my eyes. I let the sounds of the jungle in, I let my breathing settle, along with my thoughts.

'Write a book', I heard. 'Ok' I replied! 'I can do that', I've written a fair few before. 'A collaboration' I heard. 'Ok...I've done that too'. I was listening. 'With fifty women!' I heard next and my eyes flashed open. Source had my attention. 'Ok fifty women...' I said out loud 'and they all have to be over fifty'.

Fifty women over fifty. I liked that...all writing about what they've learned, documenting their wisdom. Every book collaboration I write, benefits Bali Street Mums. I've been working with their founder Kim Farr for three years already and I champion her charity. They rescue women and children from the dangers of begging on the streets of Bali's hectic tourist areas. So, I concluded, in that candle-lit meditation, that this book of women with a voice, should be dedicated to those without one...the women and children who live on the streets here.

I sent a voice mail to Kim their founder and there I had it. 'A Woman's Voice is a Revolution' was born...all proceeds going to fifty brave and courageous women and little girls here, who are supported by this very small, unique and transparent charity. One woman or child, for every year of my life...an English woman who was brought up with safety, schooling, a bedroom of her own, travel, experiences abroad to figure out who she was, time to figure out her voice. For every year of THAT life, I wanted to do something for a woman or child who had none of those opportunities.

I just needed my authors. I put a call-out on social media for fifty women over fifty to write with me...on New Years Eve...potentially the worst day in the social calendar to put a call-out for a book collaboration!

Overnight, as we entered 2023, I had half my authors. A fortnight later, we were full. We were on. And in March, we started writing.

On my laptop now rests the final manuscript of a book written by fifty remarkable women, each sharing their life wisdom, a rich tapestry of love woven with carefully crafted words and insights. They are travellers, scholars of politics, religion and science. We have a doctor, a monk, medicine carriers, mothers, journalists, grandmothers, singers, artists.

Their stories are courageous, bold and honest. They delve into their most personal of experiences. They write about becoming mothers, becoming strong, becoming spiritual, coping with loved ones who chose to die by suicide, they write about their financial freedom, sacred sensuality and sexuality. They write about the harshest truths they had to face, the harshest lies they had to burden and how they got through those dark nights.

There are hidden messages for you through this entire book, lacing every page, there are positive messages of love, abundance and support. These women, who you will likely never meet, collectively, actively and consciously, wrote just for you.

Their narratives of course, go much deeper than what we could fit into these pages. Their trials are many, from overcoming abuse, attempted suicides, alcoholism, near-death experiences, surviving unsafe relationships and abusive marriages. Their joys soar higher as they have embraced life after divorce, awakenings to their sexual fantasies; experiencing for the first-time delicious orgasms. They have found solace in the stillness of meditation and untamed depths in the midst of wild, plant medicine ceremonies.

For these women, healing has been a process of journaling, writing, talking, taking natural medicine, leaning on wise elders, girlfriends and frivolous days off from every-day life.

Our collective experiences amount to over 3,500 years of wisdom on this beautiful planet. We have birthed 82 children and 30 grandchildren. Our authors here are beautiful souls who were born to right wrongs. These women were born to herald the rise of the feminine and across the globe, their voices are being raised so you can follow.

As you turn these pages, may you feel the warmth of a 'mother figure's' hug, sage advice to lean on when you're struggling and a reassuring voice whispering, 'We have your back!'.

Each author has spoken with heartfelt sincerity, revealing intimate and previously untold stories with an authenticity that touched my soul as I carefully edited every line with them.

Each story is the truth of the woman who wrote it, recognising in their maturity that others living the same experiences, had their truth too. In speaking their personal truth, let them encourage you to speak yours.

May the energy of every story wash love over you, cleansing you, breathing new life into your spirit.

These are your sisters, your elders, your mentors—women who know what you're going through, because they've been there too.

As you dip into this sacred book of secrets, may you find solace, strength and a reminder of the resilient, radiant woman you are.

Welcome to our revolution.

@thelynetteallen
@balistreetmums-project
www.balistreetmums.org

Late-blossoming silver model,
self-confessed show-off,
embracing her age and all that goes with it!

FOREWORD
BY DEBORAH DARLING

From the moment I heard about the concept of this book, I loved the idea of fifty women over fifty sharing their wisdom. Becoming fifty was such a watershed point for me, I feel I only started to discover myself at that age.

I lost my mother when I was young, so I wasn't able to learn from her wisdom as I embarked on my own adult life. I have always had older women friends in my life, whom I looked up to and learned from. They became my guideposts.

As older women, it's so important that we share our stories. This book will be such an important source of inspiration and comfort simply because the women here have been bold enough to write their truths. Becoming a model in my fifties and using this time in my life to publicly show my age with pride, I feel my efforts are working most when young women tell me they want to be like me when they grow up! Most of us breathe in the media's lie of beauty being laughter-line free. We're meant to believe that women have children, live lives, work, have careers, go through divorces, death and illness...all without evidence of it showing on their faces or bodies – it is utter nonsense. The real shape of a woman is evidence of her life; her curves, her confidence, her laughter, her trust in her own individuality and, as a result, her unwavering sense of self!

Young women need to see older women as the wise seers and carriers of strength they are. They need to see us silver-haired beauties, the strong, capable role models we truly are, so they can find themselves post their own half century mark.

I remember the first time I saw an older woman with silver hair being depicted as attractive, stylish and uber cool in a magazine. That photo made such a huge impact on me. It was a photo of Beatrix Ost. I was just approaching fifty, I'd just received some less than flattering comments about entering my new 'fifty' era... Beatrix must have been in her early seventies at the time. I needed to see her flamboyance, her style, her personality...in print, right there in a glossy magazine, in order for me to understand how I could present my own Self!

I feel the women in this book have done the same, by writing their stories and imparting their infectious enthusiasm for life and growth.

We're all on our growing journeys, we need to know that other women have been through difficulties too. There is a message for every woman on every page of this book, a message that will find her heart and let her know she is not alone.

My own story has never seemed particularly amazing to me, it all happened so step-by-step, it was really a natural progression – one thing led to another and now here I am - so I am always thrilled to find that my ideas, words, images and courage to 'be seen' resonates with so many other women, of all ages.

It just goes to show that there's magic in ordinary stories, that there is encouragement in knowing that none of us have it all figured out, that we all still have questions. I believe that the wise words of a woman, found at just the right time, can have a profound influence on another woman's course of life.

If I could impart one of the most valuable lessons, I would say, 'Do it scared!'. I used to think that being afraid was a warning sign not to try something. I now know it's the very reason I should do something! When someone says 'fear holds you back', I genuinely didn't know that fear would 'hold me back', I thought it was a sensible red flag for me not do something - actually, it's the opposite. Fear is why you should be doing it!

Assess everything you think you know to be true and be prepared to unlearn a lot of it. Try new things, switch your routine. Walk a different route, accept invitations you wouldn't usually and engage in conversations with people of different ages and viewpoints. Discombobulate your habitual wiring and allow that to challenge your views. You'll see a different perspective and from that vantage point, new paths become visible.

When I was younger, I never imagined that I might use the wisdom I'd acquired over the years to inspire others. Yet, through my photoshoots, my voice on social media and the carefully chosen brands I work with, I have seen and continue to feel my impact.

Allow yourself to have an impact too, use your voice, flirt a little with life, the camera, yourself, let the world see and hear you, for you too, my darling, are a revolution.

@deborah_darling

In Sacred Eldership order
...we begin

Our elder in this book, it's been her friends and clients over the years who have encouraged her to use her voice.

As a mother and grandmother, she's had to advocate for herself and those she loves. As an artist, a teacher, a designer, director, creator and fundraiser, she's used her voice to create, inspire, motivate and educate.

With her words in this book, she's ready to co-create a revolution!

KATE PEACE

WRITE IT ALL DOWN

One of the amazing gifts I've brought from my childhood and my first marriage, when there were no meaningful conversations or sharing of hopes, dreams or fears, is the ability to communicate very clearly by writing it down.

Back then, it became apparent that my husband and I didn't have any time or space in our relationship to talk (being highly committed to demanding projects) and I realised he had a reluctance to discussing 'emotional' relationship issues or potentially 'upsetting' topics. My wonderful generous, loving partner, who would do anything for me found 'sharing', both a waste of time and 'unproductive'.

He is however, a writer. He loves words. So, my first innovation was to write him a letter about how I felt. I wrote simply and unemotionally (I read it through several times to check for clarity and had a good friend do the same).

He read it and instantly understood my point of view. Initiating 'conversation' was trickier. The eventual solution, was for my husband to write a journal page every day, for our eyes only!

He has now done this every morning ever since, whilst I meditate. He writes what's on his mind, he writes about his dreams, memories and more and more often, about how much and why he loves me!

These precious pages....twenty-five years of them...have initiated great conversation, conversations that begin with his words. Particularly since he retired, this has been a true and long standing heart-filled 'sharing'.

PASS IT ON

A few years ago, just in time for my eight-first birthday, I qualified as an Ayurvedic Practitioner and as with all my passions...Art, Textiles, Tai Chi, Chi Gung, Yoga, Meditation, Ling Chi Healing, I pass that knowledge on.

I've always wanted to learn as much as I could in order to pass it on to others; ever since the first time I experienced the truly unselfish urge to give back, in 1956 during the profound revelations of art education.

For me, it feels similar to the joyous feeling that comes when you've seen a fantastically moving film or just read an extraordinarily enchanting book and you know just the person who'd love it.

Like all the best avenues of teaching, learning never comes to an end; in the passing of information forwards and in the teaching of it, I'm always assured of new vistas opening up. I'm witness to constant miracles of the human being's capacity for healing and I delight in new relationships with people I'd never have met otherwise.

As I immerse myself of late, in the healing powers of Ayurvedic Medicine, imagine the sheer bliss of being with someone as they discover their own healing power and gain new strength, courage, awareness, fulfilment or peace.

I cannot think of anything I would rather be doing in my final decades. My Dharma has at last found me!

THERE'S A GIFT IN EVERY WOUND

I feel now that my capacity to see what I've learned through each wound, is getting faster. I see more clearly why my inner Self and Spirit, put me through the fires it did.

It was four decades before I could forgive my Mother; for what I've considered blighting my life and ruining past relationships. During a silent retreat some years later, I was able to ask her forgiveness and really feel gratitude to her for bringing me into this world against terrible and tragic odds.

I started to appreciate the many gifts she gave me. My passion for everything in life was born from experiencing scarcity. It developed out of having to 'create something from nothing', which she had done as I watched. I remember her making clothes for me from second hand army uniforms and silk parachutes after the war for instance.

Seeing the gifts after my first marriage ended, took a mere twelve years! And when a decade ago, I was given a diagnosis of Osteoarthritis and offered pain killers, for what were by then, painful, partially useless hands, I found and fully engaged with Ayurvedic philosophy, the healing treatment of Panchakarma and the wonderful art of Mudra...not only to heal my hands but also to heal my life!

When you can shift your perspective and ask yourself the question 'If there IS something to be learned in this situation, what is it?'. I've often asked, 'Why would my Spirit (who is always trying to move me towards healing), give me this?'.

As always, I find such dialogues are even more creative when shared with a friend, who can offer a new way of seeing things. Even drawing an oracle card when you're on your own or in meditation, just sitting quietly, can bring answers and help you see the gift in your wounds.

KEEP HYDRATED

About twelve years ago, as I was getting interested in learning more about the practices of Ayurveda, a friend fresh from a weekend course, offered me a 'magic' drink from her flask.

It smelled so fragrant as she poured it. I found it delicious, refreshing and comforting. And when I learned the benefits, I was really hooked!

Often known as 'Tissue Water' because both the presence of plant nutrients and the warmth of the liquid make it easily assimilated by the body's many layers of tissue, I experienced this for myself over the next few weeks. I infused the spices (coriander, cumin and fennel) in water just off the boil and drank it daily instead of water.

The texture of my skin improved, as did my digestion and quality of sleep and I felt generally much more relaxed.

I've been drinking Tissue Water daily ever since, I feel fully hydrated even though I'm drinking less than before...this 'tea' certainly knows its way around the body!

CONSIDER A RELATIONSHIP CONTRACT

About forty years ago I met Brian, at first a friend; he helped me find my feet after I'd left my first marriage. Some years on, when it seemed we could be in a relationship, we acknowledged our fears of being hurt. His fear was more to do with commitment, his preference was for an 'open' relationship and I wanted commitment and sexual fidelity. I also wanted a space where we could face, resolve and grow from our differences.

A Quantity Surveyor at the time, he was used to the idea of 'renewable contracts', where he might hire a building firm on a short contract for example. So, I suggested that we have a short three-six month contract, which we could amend, renew or end by mutual discussion and agreement.

He liked the idea! So, we created a list of nine agreements, to support each other in following our soul paths whether we personally liked them or not. They've worked so well, all nine of them, we still love these agreements and actually...we got married in the end and are celebrating our thirty-third wedding anniversary!

Take a stand to feel refreshed in overwhelm or stress

When life lays me low or I feel overwhelmed or indecisive, I've learned to change my state by how I stand, breathe or behave.

Sometimes, I'll take a pause, stop what I'm doing and breathe in and out deeply for a few full breaths, exhaling with a growl or even a roar, a scream or a yelp, whatever I think will make me feel better at the time! I release what I need to in the moment.

Other times I stand like a force of nature (imagining myself as a tree, rock or a mountain) and I close my eyes. I plant my feet firmly in the ground (even better when I stand, not on carpet but on the earth outside) and, as I breathe in, I lift my body, standing tall, creating space between all my joints, especially the spine. I bring my chin towards my chest, lengthening the back of my neck and I feel a pull from my crown towards to sky and the heavens, as if I'm connecting to a star.

In these moments, I feel connected both to Heaven and Earth, the two great cosmic powers, I breathe in Yin energy from the ground and Yang energy from the sky. I feel like it refreshes the energy in all my cells, 'just like recharging a battery' my Chi Gung teacher used to say.

Such mindful moments have made the world of difference to me, really allowing a reset, a change in perspective or an energy boost, as refreshing as a cold shower, in less than a minute!

Life is a work of art

Although I no longer work as a professional artist, I use the principles of art every day, in all I do. Over sixty years ago, I learned that art is about 'co-creating' with the medium available to me. I've navigated life in the same way, with the materials I have...my characteristics, my needs and my personality. They all respond more creatively when they're listened to.

Every morning I co-create myself, in the best possible image I can. Just like I did with art...now I use ritual, intention, breath, movement and prayer to awaken my cells into a world of love and light.

Sometimes I add in some of the energy medicine I've learned and I've found that journaling, gratitude and visualising, really lift my spirits, helping my trillions of cells renew themselves. I think of this as my first 'Act of Power' of the day. Spending time with myself on my own in this way makes such a difference to me.

I feel this improves my health, I have energy to face the day and I feel happier and healthier now at eighty-two years of age, than I did thirty years ago.

Re-name, re-christen or re-birth yourself

It was literally a defining moment for me. In 1956 having recently started an Art Degree Course, my new friends and I fervently agreed that the name 'Beryl' (my christened name), despite being a precious gem in the gate of Heaven, just wasn't appropriate for who I was becoming.

I disliked it intensely as a child and as soon as I left home, I changed my name to Kate. I really loved the crisp, self-made sound. Changing my name embodied the severing of some childhood traumas too, it changed the way I saw myself and the way others saw me.

I never forgot that power of re-naming, re-shaping and re-telling my story...no longer through a victim's lens of poverty and neglect but from a place of 'anything's possible'.

Looking back, it's been fascinating to see how many times I've reframed situations, relationships or social conventions to create a life I love. That possibility was born in me when my circle of friends gave me the confidence to re-christen and rebirth myself!

An elder in guardianship of ancient rituals and practices, she holds herself accountable for her voice, her words, her deeds and behaviours.

As a daughter, she was her mother's voice when her wishes needed to be heard at her fathers bedside in hospital. As a mother, she stood up for her two children when the education system seemed to think they knew what was best for them and now she uses her wise words sparingly.

Often in silence, in her Red Shed, she is called upon more and more to use her voice and wise words in the opening of medicine and healing ceremonies across the world. Soak up her words, you will find comfort in them.

@visionarysagecrone

SALLIE WARMAN-WATTS

FEAR IS ONLY CONTAINED IN THE MIND

"You are a fucking legend, mother!' my forty-eight-year-old son told me. Some time ago, I decided I needed to sample all that life has to offer...including those aspects of life that were supposedly wrong or deemed bad for me!

I am walking my path of self-discovery and part of this has involved plant medicine. At the tender age of seventy, I sat in Ceremony with Mother Ayahuasca, Grandfather San Pedro and the heart-opening plant medicine Sassafras in a beautiful week-long deep-dive connection with myself.

During these journeys with the teacher plants, I learned much about who I am, how I have been formed into the woman I am today and how to turn fear of the unknown into a strength. Over this period, it occurred to me that I hadn't wanted to confide my sacred path or my plant medicine journeys with my children. Why should that be?

After some thought, I realised it might well be fear...fear of judgement, fear of them losing respect for me, fear of losing their love, fear of them seeing the woman in me rather than their mother.

What have I really learned then? That 'fear' is only in the contained mind of someone yet to believe in themselves. For when confronting my fear through conversations with my children regarding my actions, they fully released me from my own guilt and fear of rejection, by allowing me to break out of that contained mind.

So, as you can guess, I told my son, "I do believe, I am a fucking legend".

HEAL THE MOTHER WOUND

The mother wound - a cultural and ancestral trauma passed down through generations, it is rained upon daughters by their mothers, who in turn, can go on to wound their own children. Harsh but true.

We're talking about it though and many are breaking the cycle. It sounds and looks like an obvious realised behaviour to break but it can be so subtle and insidious, often we are oblivious to its cuts. I've experienced it as a daughter, lived unknowingly with it and then in turn, I passed it on to mine.

I can tell you, this dawning was painful. But I'm breaking the cycle and vowing that the wounding in my own family ends here, with me. And maybe, because you're reading this, it ends in your family too.

In my vow, I say this...for me, to be a mother, is to be humble. I will listen and be non-judgemental, I will drop into my heart space, as hard as it might be when I feel the justification of hurt and I will stop. I will remember that the final part of the giving of myself to you, the daughter I birthed, is more important.

It is our daughters that are the future, not us. Their experiences of the world are shown through us and our actions. To cry together and be vulnerable together, when as a mother, you think your heart will break because you can't bear to hear any more of your perceived imperfections, means to hold on tighter. The end is in sight, as forgiveness is about to enter the arena.

Daughters...when we accept who our mothers really were or are, forgiveness is available. Mothers...try not to judge your daughters, keep your heart open and emotionally available to climb every mountain with her, together, forever.

THIS TOO SHALL PASS

During a time in my life, when all seemed dark and there was no 'light at the end of the tunnel', a deep knowing blinked every now and again, like a buoy out at sea. You know the ones, when you're staring out to sea into that inky black night and you think you see a light flickering. You stare harder, hoping you're not mistaken and that there truly is a light, far out on the horizon.

That brave light standing alone, is the symbol of all that you're holding: hope. The anchor in the storm. The guiding light to safety. The beacon that draws you home.

When both my parents died, a short time apart, I was adrift, drowning, I couldn't see the light. Then one day, when I managed to raise myself from my bed, I sat in front of my mirror. Stuck to it was a post-it note, 'This too Shall Pass', it read. I bowed my head and cried. I knew the sincerity of those words to be true. I carried my body from room to room that morning and in each room I visited, I found more post-it notes attached to furniture or walls declaring 'This too shall pass'. Slowly, I began to understand why this beautiful man I called my husband had placed them in each room.

In his desperation to heal my heart, these words were his only solace, his buoy, his guiding light to my way back home. So as each day, each week, each month passed, I found the truth and beauty in these words. You know, the only constant in this world is change my love. Whatever you're going through 'This too shall pass'.

LOVE YOURSELF

I want to tell you that I know exactly what love is but I can't. I want to tell you how to feel love but I can't. I want to tell you how to find love but I can't.

I've lived this long, I should be able to tell you all about love but all I can do, is tell you the way I love. My belief is that there are many ways to love, loving a man, a woman, a child, our parents, friends or love for an animal, an object, our planet Earth. I love with my heart wide open, with my eyes wide open, with my body wide open and with my soul wide open.

I have been hurt of course and briefly, it has stopped me but in all these seventy years, I've learned that my heart mends, it repairs quickly if I just let it just BE and that enables me to go on and love again just as fiercely.

I'm a passionate woman, in all areas of my life and love is no different. There's also no difference in who I love, for if I love you, whomever you are, you have all of me, every drop of my being, for all of my life. There are no conditions, no judgements, no limits. When I learned to love myself, completely, it was easier to love others.

I think if you love yourself, you don't need the love of others to sustain you, you can do that for yourself, therefore freeing you unconditionally to love, whoever you feel called to.

I suppose the answers to the questions are;

What is love: it's you
How to feel love: feel you
How to find love: inside you

LOVE IS YOU every time.

YOUR PAST DOES NOT DEFINE YOU DARLING

As I sat staring out of my window one day, with the rain trickling down the pane, like tears leaving my eyes and falling onto my cheeks, I asked myself the question 'Am I the sum total of my past? Is this who I really am?'. I glanced over my shoulder as if looking down through the annals of time to remember.
In a land that time forgot...

I forgot I took the first contraceptive Pill
I forgot I could not get a mortgage by myself
I forgot I needed my husband's permission to open a bank account
I forgot childbirth was silent and, on my back,
I forgot that sexual harassment was normal
I forgot I lived in sin with my first love, not married
I forgot pregnancy out of wedlock was a sin
I forgot abortions were illegal
I forgot that divorce was not a choice for a woman
I forgot that depression was frowned upon
I forgot that menopause and periods were a dirty secret
I forgot that marital rape was allowed
I forgot that children should be seen and not heard
I forgot domestic abuse was my fault
I had forgotten so much of importance and yet...

Through all this, I never forgot myself and I will never forget my own sovereignty. Adversity is my power and my wisdom.

But is this really me? Yes and no, it's part of me. I am who I am because I've been through what I have. Life has touched me but not tainted me. Life will touch you, don't allow it to taint you.

RELEASE YOUR CHILDREN

In recent years, I began to grow into myself, the autonomy of who I am, the pushing back against the old paradigms of who I thought I was. It had an unexpected knock-on effect, it began to stimulate that part of me that yearned for freedom. The dawning of the concept of 'consensual release' has been liberating.

I needed to let go of my children, in order for me and them to fly or I'd have always been nesting and never found time in my life for me, which could well have been a slow suffocating duty of responsibility.

This 'consensual release' came when I realised they were safe, when I realised they'd got this, when I realised they'd got their lives and their hearts sorted (or something that resembled it!) and I stopped needing them emotionally myself. When I knew I was becoming fully grown into my own skin (not as a mother or a wife) but as the single human I started out as, the woman I aspired to be (with her dreams and desires, before conditioning and peer pressure took hold) emerged.

The guilt disappeared, emotional pressure was released and replaced by the tender loving mutual respect and the independent, sovereign, ME that emerged. I have only recently realised that the part of myself which was my own expansion, the deep need of expansiveness of my mind, body and soul, came because I released myself from my own emotional need of my children!

Wow! This has been a huge lesson for me. I have sat with this for a while. Almost like breast feeding, our babies stimulate our milk to flow, so too does being close to them. And when your body and mind cry out for separation from this emotional need to be responsible, way past their need for us, somehow mothers want to cling on.

But in that consensual release, we emerge and life itself blossoms, so that in the end, our life's work of nurturing provider falls into completeness and absolute certainty of the heartfelt wholeness of motherhood, it is done. And you, you are free to be you. Enjoy!

YOU DON'T HAVE TO 'HEAL' ALL THE TIME, LIFE IS FOR LIVING TOO

As we journey through life, we live all kinds of emotions and experiences. Sometimes joyful, sometimes painful, sometimes traumatic. When we go through our perception of trauma, we develop trauma responses and coping strategies. We often feel the need to 'heal', to bring our responses back into balance once the traumatic event itself has passed.

The pain from trauma can be alleviated; accepting trauma for what it was doesn't mean it disappears. Unless we erase the memories or block it completely, any experience we've lived, can and will always remain but we can manage our response to it better through various healing modalities. And then...we need to move on.

Too much emphasis on healing and seeing our 'shadow selves' isn't healthy either. You are not broken. Don't spend so much of your time 'healing' that you forget to live. It can be so emotionally draining, that work and while you're focused on the past, you're taking away from the life you're living now...all the best bits are passing you by.

Too much navel gazing can cause upset in itself. Take respite, see the light at the end of the tunnel, take a rest from all the angst!

IMAGINE RELEASING ALL THAT CONTAINS YOU, IMAGINE WHAT FREEDOM LOOKS LIKE FOR A WOMAN

Would it be so inconceivable for a woman to be totally free from 'containment'? Because contained is what we have always been. We have always belonged to others, as daughters, wives, mothers, colleagues, friends... slaves even to our bodies.

Imagine for a moment, what releasing all that containment would look like...freedom to just 'be'...standing in your own sovereignty, the expansiveness within your heart and soul, free from guilt.

I began to realise something was shifting within my being after meditating with ceremonial cacao, I started four years ago in my mid-sixties. Ceremonial cacao is a heart-opening plant medicine. Taken in its raw form, it contains Theobroma. We meditate after drinking it in ritual and changes in our understanding of who we are, can emerge.

I became aware and also open, to other plant medicines. They started to teach me the ways of the heart, the soul and infinite consciousness. The more I grew, the more I was able to let go of old paradigms.

Sit for a moment in stillness and tell yourself 'I am truly free', allow yourself a no-barriers/only trust approach. Try to carry no guilt in this process and instead, think 'freedom' and feel 'love'. Practice this daily. You'll begin to feel the expansiveness of the Universe growing inside you, the power that is you and yes, freedom will emerge.

Life will touch you,
don't allow it to taint you

Her mother, Margaret Golding and the powerful women in her family helped her find her voice, along with her dear friend Catherine who died in her 99th year.

As a child, she always stood up for those who couldn't stand up for themselves. One of ten children, she learned early on to use her voice to be heard.

Believing in herself and cultivating presence has been a powerful tool for her, perhaps more powerful than her words.

Her wish to become an author and collaborate with other women, came true in this book!

@inspiredmindcoaching

PHILOMENA JORDAN-PATRIKIOS

FILL YOUR LIFE WITH POWERFUL WOMEN MENTORS

Catherine died a few days after her ninety-ninth birthday. Intelligent, stoic and strong, she not only shared these traits with my own beautiful mother, who held the same Irish lineage but she also became like a second mother to me when I met her in my eleventh year.

I've been blessed with powerful female role models throughout my life; women who had a fiery streak and seemed to know their worth intuitively. They've come in various ages, cultures, shapes and sizes. Women who have often endured suffering, injustice and tragedy in their lives and yet have found a way to transform their suffering into strength, the injustice into integrity and the tragedy into compassion.

All have left an indelible mark on my soul, sharing lessons from their own history, inspiring me to explore other avenues and ways of thinking and being.

"Let it be." Catherine called out one day, quoting from the Beatle's song, as we sat together sipping freshly poured tea in beautiful china cups, munching on home-made cake. "Let it be," she repeated, "it's the answer to a happy life". She beamed as she said it. Such a simple truth.

Whenever I'm in need of a simple truth, I turn to the wisdom of the women gone before me, the sisterhood currently in my life and those yet to come.

I encourage you to surround yourself with powerful women, whether in real life or in books and podcasts. Fill your soul with their wisdom gleaned from lives of challenge and joy, so that you may fill others in turn.

FOLLOW YOUR BREATH TO DECLUTTER YOUR MIND

As beings of consciousness, we each have the choice to stagnate or grow, to stay stuck in the past or to expand in our knowledge and awareness. I say that now with the wisdom of age but in my younger years, I floated through life with little sense of time or purpose.

It was as though I was standing on the side-lines rather than co-creating in the choreography of life's dance.

I used to dream of having a magic machine that, at the press of a button, could answer any of my many questions about life, instead, I had to rely on the Encyclopaedia Britannica and my local library. Today, that magic machine (the internet) is here, providing me with journeys to the cosmos, sitting with and listening to amazing minds sharing their wisdom on a myriad of subjects. However, I'm becoming more discerning about how much more I put into my head and for what purpose.

What if, as my Buddhist teachers remind me, all one really needs to know, is already within? What if the accumulation of knowledge becomes an addiction? Like the accumulation of furniture, clothes or things that clutter our homes...so much so that new storage units have been created to house our overflow!

What about the overflow in our minds? Just as decluttering the house allows one to move more freely, with more ease and satisfaction, so too can decluttering the mind. It brings spaciousness where one can sit in stillness and silence, perhaps travelling within where the wisdom truly lies.

You don't have to sit for hours. Just one or two minutes of simply following and counting the breath as it flows into the nostrils and out from the nostrils; one minute of staying present with the breath, is enough to bring a sigh of relief and thus the decluttering process in the mind can begin.

CULTIVATE AN ATTITUDE OF GRATITUDE

Gratitude is among the highest of elevated emotions. Having kept gratitude journals for the past fifteen years, I live in a state of thankfulness most of the time.

At first, I found writing in a journal really challenging, so I began slowly. I wrote the date on the page and just three things I was grateful for, using the simple template: 'I am grateful for.... because...'.

I stalled so many times thinking I needed to write about amazing things but I soon saw that the tiny things evoked feelings of gratitude for me: walking the dog, seeing a rainbow, finding a white feather. While it only takes a few moments to write these short sentences, the secret is to rest into the feeling of being grateful.

For me, journalling at bedtime, means my body can benefit all night from the feel-good hormones that gratitude induces. Over time, I've realised that while it's easy to be grateful for all that's positive, there's something profound about finding gratitude in the difficulties that can assail us all. In learning to be grateful to people and situations that challenged me, I began to notice subtle changes within and I don't sit with the rise of anger or other fear-based emotions for long anymore.

Through keeping a gratitude journal, I've learnt lessons about myself. I've faced my reflection in other people and situations and I've taken responsibility for my reactions.

Gratitude has helped me go beyond habitual preconceived ideas and opened me up to new perceptions. It seems the more grateful I am, the more people and situations come into my life for me to be grateful for. It's been an upward spiral and I've found it my perfect way to manifest.

All it takes is a small notebook, a pen and the intention to notice and record the good, while transmuting the bad and the ugly into powerful sensations of heart-felt gratitude.

BE MINDFUL - YOU ARE NOT YOUR THOUGHTS

It's so interesting to me, to observe the mind and the inner dialogue that can be activated so easily, particularly where my family are concerned. As one of eleven children, there were plenty of hierarchical dramas that, decades later, still echo into our relationships.

Even with years of practising mindfulness, I'm aware of the temptation to react defensively to an email or a text and I find myself rehearsing conversations that are entirely fabricated in my mind...by my mind!

Becoming aware of the thoughts and feelings that arise from these mind conversations, enables me to step back. When the email or text arrives, I know I'm likely to read it through, first from the lens of my own past experience and I catch myself. I read it again and realise how I'm translating their words through the filters I've built up over time, regarding this relationship.

I come back to the gift of 'mindfulness' and the letting go of old habitual patterns. And no, I haven't got my act completely together but I have learned to know that I am not my thoughts. I can choose what and how to think and thus respond skilfully and mindfully.

It's a gift I would gladly give to all.

KEEP STEPPING INTO YOUR POWER

Old habits are never far away, ready to drag me two steps back. Even at this age and with all my experience of life, doubt arises and it's my destroyer of action if I entertain it for too long.

In times like this, I use Oracle Cards for wisdom and guidance. I shuffled my pack of medicine cards recently and the card 'Antelope' sprang forth. The message was 'Take action! Do it now!'.

Well, that was about right. How easily I had slipped into the subconscious patterns of procrastination, blame and shame. Just when I needed it, Antelope taught me to get up, shake it all off and learn once again the fallibility of being human and to clearly see the challenges that self-doubt can present. The Antelope card reminded me to let go of doubt and return to that place of strength within. It was as though he was whispering to me, as a loving mother might whisper to her beloved child,

> 'You have strayed from the path. Have compassion on yourself - you have
> come a long way. These challenges have arisen that you might push beyond
> your self-imposed boundaries and into new territory. You know that's how it works'

I felt that inner strength nudge me forward and I stepped, anew, into my power.

BE THE CHANGE YOU WISH TO SEE

 Charles Dickens wrote 'It was the best of times, it was the worst of times' in 1859; I feel it's an apt description of the world today and which version I adhere to, depends on my perspective in that moment.

Quantum physics tells me that everything is energy and that energy flows where attention goes. If I keep my focus on what's going wrong, I feel I add to the denser frequency of fear and the world looks like a scary place. However, with the spotlight on the amazing people and events happening all around me, I sense a move into the higher frequencies of love and the world becomes a heaven on earth.

I believe that more people are awakening to the concept that 'we create our own reality', which may bring about a change from a victimhood mentality to becoming the author of our own destiny.

I feel the speed at which change is taking place is both exciting and unnerving. We seem to be reaching a pinnacle in history where we can, individually and collectively, choose to make the shift into oneness rather than separation, love rather than fear.

I, for one, am glad to be alive at this moment in time. The call to you dear reader, from me, is to be the change you wish to see in the world and the world will change accordingly. With the rise of feminine energy moving us towards inner peace and freedom, I believe each one of us is being invited to usher in the very best of times.

LET YOUR VOICE BE HEARD

Your voice is an instrument in the symphony of life. A child sings for the joy of hearing their own voice. They don't judge the sounds they create, they just create...humming and singing, their cells resonating, bringing harmony and balance.

Science is catching up with what Indigenous traditions have known for thousands of years, that sound can soothe and literally heal us on a cellular level. Throughout my life, my voice has been a reflection of my emotions. Loud and boisterous in younger years, wanting to be heard, then hoarse and hurt when misunderstood. My voice would splinter with the crashing sea waves and be hurled back at me by mighty winds as I stood on giant rocks, releasing whatever was crying out to be released. That same voice was small and muffled as I cried with shame and confusion into pillows of loneliness and grief.

All those years, unable to express what was deep inside of me for fear of being judged, I spoke words that covered my fear like a cloak of confidence that few could see through. The cloak was removed gently by a wise mentor that I finally confided in. Sharing one's truth with a friend, a mentor or coach, can free the song that is waiting to be heard. Now, from this place of alignment in my sixty-eighth year, I use my voice to speak my truth and sing to my heart's content.

So, let your voice be an instrument of encouragement for others. Let your voice be an instrument of peace. Let your voice be an instrument of love, soothing hurts and fears. Sing, hum, chant, speak up, speak loud, speak soft; use your voice and be heard...

It's never too late to start over

As I approached my sixtieth birthday, a colleague joked about 'retirement' age and something clicked in my mind. Looking back on my life, I realised that I had always dreamed of owning a wellbeing studio and establishing my own coaching practice. With retirement on the horizon, I decided to take action and make my dreams a reality.

I had lived a life full of adventure, following my heart first to France and then to Greece, immersing myself in two very different cultures and languages. Then came the middle years of motherhood, marriage and teaching, when I struggled to juggle everything and beat myself up when I fell short. However, I had also accumulated a wealth of knowledge from self-help courses and modalities that I later found useful in building my own business. As I trusted my instincts and set the wheels in motion, more people and opportunities showed up for me.

Six years ago, I was lucky enough to acquire a studio in a beautiful converted church where I had facilitated meditation and mindfulness. Thus was born my own coaching practice and it all fell into place.

Now at sixty-eight, I wake up excited every day, doing what I'm passionate about; coaching incredible people who inspire me as they go from feeling stuck to making their own breakthroughs. Of course, life still presents challenges but I view them as growth opportunities and I feel privileged to be living the life I've always wanted.

Take a chance on something new, remember that it's never too late to make a brand-new start.

A mother and grandmother, an inquisitive traveller, she says so many people have supported her to use her voice, one of the most prominent being her first mentor, Anthony Robbins!

She speaks out on her own weekly radio show these days and sings loudly in Kirtan.

As DJ Chica, her voice guides people into the deepest and most moving of internal journeys during ecstatic dance ceremonies, which she hosts all over the globe!

@prelovedchica

ELENE MARSDEN

AFTER BEREAVEMENT, FIND THE GRATITUDE

When I met my husband, we were just teenagers, full of youthful energy and promise. He was determined to spend his life with me and I was swept off my feet by his devotion. He said many times that he would spend his life with me and he kept his promise! For forty-six amazing years, we shared a rich and fulfilling life together, we raised three wonderful sons and created a lifetime of memories.

But when he was diagnosed with cancer, everything changed. It was a devastating blow. Watching him battle the disease was one of the toughest things I've ever experienced. He finally passed away after six short months and I was left heartbroken and lost.

But even in my darkest moments, I knew I had to keep going. I remembered the journey we'd planned together, a trip to Japan to visit our son and I decided to take the trip on my own. It was scary to venture out into the world without my partner by my side but I was determined to make it happen.

My journey included a four-day boat trip from Osaka to Shanghai, passing by the many islands and bridges that my husband had loved so much, I felt his presence with me and I cried. I travelled through six different countries over the course of sixty days and I began to heal. I shared my story with others and found solace in their empathy and understanding. I knew I was lucky to have experienced so much love in my life and that his love would always be with me.

Grief is a natural emotion which changes over time. I will always miss him and I'm grateful for the love and the memories. The poet Dylan Thomas wrote so eloquently, "Though lovers be lost, love shall not".

If you're experiencing loss, take a moment to feel gratitude for the love that still surrounds you, love of family, friends, partners, even pets. Cherish that and let it nurture you.

SAY YES

A few years back, I visited friends in Maspalomas, a breath-taking place with miles of sandy dunes. I planned this trip to coincide with the anniversary of my husband's passing and on the anniversary, as the sun rose, I climbed to the top of the highest sand dune, where we'd both been before. I remember my husband, a black belt karate teacher, running up those dunes like a teenager, despite his illness. In his memory, I lit a candle, some incense and let the sounds of the ocean waves wash over me, giving thanks for the love we shared.

As the morning passed, people started arriving on the beach below me...some dressed...many naked. It's a naturist beach, you see and I'm not sure why but in that moment, I wanted to feel free, liberated and to prove to myself that I could make my own decisions and experience life as fully as they were.

With perfect weather and just a few days left before leaving the island, I knew it was now or never. I took off my top, then my shorts and walked half a mile completely naked. Feeling the wind on my body, the waves lapping at my feet, was a unique experience.

I remember that day vividly, mustering up the courage to step outside my comfort zone and take a leap of faith. To my surprise, I found unexpected joy in that experience and it reminded me of the endless possibilities that await, when we take a chance.

If not now, then when? Don't wait any longer to make your dreams a reality. Make plans, take action, you've got this!

MEDITATE EVERY SINGLE DAY

In my early twenties, I made the decision to embark on a journey of self-discovery by learning meditation. It was a natural calling, I've always had a free-spirited, hippie soul. My introduction was through Transcendental Meditation, where I was given my own personal mantra. It was an experience that has stayed with me for forty years. I've never shared my personal mantra with anyone - it's my own little secret!

Meditation has been a constant companion through all the highs and lows of life. It helped me tremendously in difficult times. Without this practice, I would have had a much harder time coping.

Nowadays, I practice chakra meditation, which directs my attention to the seven energy centres in my body but it really doesn't matter what type of meditation you choose, as long as it calms you, relaxes you and helps you be more present. If sitting still for long periods isn't your thing, a walk in nature can be just as effective.

Choose whatever works for you.

Nowadays, I practice chakra meditation, which directs my attention to the seven energy centres in my body but it really doesn't matter what type of meditation you choose, as long as it calms you, relaxes you and helps you be more present. If sitting still for long periods isn't your thing, a walk in nature can be just as effective. Choose whatever works for you.

GROW OLD DISGRACEFULLY

As I enter my mid-sixties, I feel grateful for my freedom. My children have grown up and I'm not responsible for elderly parents. I live life on my own terms and pursue my passions. I've been fortunate enough to travel to amazing destinations, make wonderful friends and contribute to my community with a weekly radio show and I volunteer for a local charity...and there's a part of me that yearns for more.

Growing up, I followed the rules and lived a conventional life. Now though, I want to break free and try new things. In the last five years, I've added excitement, sensuality and sexuality to my life. I've sung my heart out at Karaoke bars, explored my inner goddess through incredible, tantric massages and I'm enjoying intimate sexual relationships with friends who each bring something special to my life.

I know this adventurous phase won't last forever, eventually I will embrace a more serene lifestyle but for now, I'm taking risks and reaping the rewards. I've been doing some soul searching lately and it hit me...when my time comes, I want to look back on my life with no regrets. So, I'm encouraging you to do the same.

What have you always wanted to do? Don't let fear or self-doubt hold you back. It's never too late, pursue your dreams, create a life that brings you genuine happiness. Trust me, it's worth it!

FIND YOUR REASON FOR BEING

Ikigai is a beautiful Japanese concept meaning 'your reason for being'. It's all about finding your life purpose, your ultimate bliss. For me, that bliss is Ecstatic Dance. I discovered it during the pandemic while living in Bali.

Every Friday and Sunday morning, I would gather with others to freestyle dance in the spiritual capital of Ubud. The music was incredible, I felt so free moving to those beautiful rhythms with no constraints. I loved everything about it - the rituals, the DJ's music, the journey of self-discovery and the relaxing shivasana pose at the end.

I decided to learn DJ skills so I could offer Ecstatic Dance to my community back in the UK, bringing a small piece of exotic Bali back to Suffolk.

It took twenty days of hard work and training to learn the art of DJing but I did it, I hosted my first Ecstatic Dance event when I got back home. I was nervous but it turned out to be a huge success! For a whole year, I hosted regular dances for a growing crowd of followers. Together, we released emotions, became more empowered as we danced our joy within a really supportive community. Last year, I travelled with my kit and DJ'd in Tokyo, Thailand and Saudi Arabia! Everywhere I went, people encouraged me to host more events. I knew I'd found my Ikigai.

Just two years ago, I would never have imagined becoming a DJ, let alone an international one! I go by the name DJ Chica, which in Spanish means 'girl' - a pretty outlandish name for a sixty-five-year-old grandma! It's easy to get caught up in the limitations society places on us based on age but let me tell you, age is nothing but a number, don't let anyone tell you otherwise!

Don't hold back, even if your dreams seem far-fetched, this is your life we're talking about and we get one shot at it. Don't waste any more time, go out there, chase your dreams and make every moment count!

STRIKE A 'POWER POSE'

One of my favourite life hacks for feeling strong, is to strike a 'power pose'. Whenever I need to prepare for a tough meeting or an important conversation, I stand with my hands on my hips, feet shoulder-width apart and hold it for a minute. It helps me feel more confident and prepared and the effects last way beyond the pose itself.

Even just thinking about these poses can help you feel stronger! Let your body take the shape of a confident, powerful stance. Use your mind to focus on feelings of strength and capability. If you repeat the phrase 'I am powerful', you'll feel more powerful in your daily life.

If you need a little extra self-care, try the self-hug pose. Give yourself a gentle embrace, it's a soothing and cathartic way to show yourself some love, when you're feeling vulnerable or unresourceful.

Think of these poses as tools. Moving your body shifts your emotional state and empowers you to take on any challenge that comes your way. Go ahead and strike that power pose!

TRAVEL...JUST DO IT

As a child, I was shy and easily frightened. A distant memory now I'm in my sixties and an adventurous world traveller but I used to be afraid of being alone and abandoned.

I want to tell you, I know now, I didn't have to be afraid. I've embraced the excitement of exploring new places on my own and I've met incredible people who reinforced my belief in the goodness of humanity. People everywhere share a love of family, friends and community...I've seen it in the markets of Beijing, I've felt it in the souks of Saudi Arabia.

I learned to let go of those fears and replace them with a sense of wonder and awe for the beauty of our planet. If you're considering a travel adventure, don't wait - start planning, there's a whole world out there waiting to be discovered.

Make plans, even if you can't go yet, planning is part of the fun...the world is brimming with fascinating cultures, stunning landscapes and exciting experiences just waiting to be explored. Take that first step towards adventure and embrace all the incredible possibilities that await you. They are there and so are the people to welcome you!

FIND YOUR VOICE AND OPEN UP!

My husband was my everything - my best friend, my partner in crime, my rock. He was always there for me, words of wisdom and guidance, we had a great relationship, I truly believed we could conquer anything together.

But then, one day, he was gone. I was devastated, completely shattered by the loss of my soulmate. For a while, I felt like life was over. I couldn't imagine going on without him. I didn't know how to deal with the overwhelming emotions that were crashing over me.

At that point, I realised I needed to delve into my emotions and start talking. Previous conversations had been so light-hearted and superficial, I'd never really let anyone see the vulnerable, raw parts of me but now, I knew I had to start opening up if I was ever going to heal.

It wasn't easy. I felt so much sadness deep inside but with friends support, I learned how to trust and open up. Through tears and heartfelt conversations, I found the words to express my feelings and discovered what truly mattered to me.

Having a support system is essential when dealing with grief and loss. We all need people to confide in, those who listen without judgment. My friends held my hand and listened to my pain, they never once made me feel like I was alone.

Cultivating those relationships takes effort but it's worth it. Let your friends know how much they mean to you – why not send a message to a friend now, thanking them for being in your life. They are a vital part of our lives and bring so much joy and comfort, especially during times of struggle.

She started to raise her voice as a traumatised 'war grandchild', sharing her journey and that of her mother and grandmother. That process connected her deeply with her inner voice and that of the ancient divine.

She's raised her voice for her spiritual Self and her children. A spokeswoman publically, she's also spoken her deepest truths privately.

"This book opens up a holy space to be inspired and heal. I'm honoured to be part of this amazing group of women!" she says.

@blooming_from_the_roots

GUDRUN OTTEN

PLAY TO CONNECT

"A soft violet rose gently opens herself to a new journey through timeless landscapes of stunning inner beauty. Scented with drops of the purest ocean side morning dew, an undestroyable fragility starts breathing you in and out, awakening those parts that are soaked with wisdom and a mystical connection to source. It is from here, where you start to become that soft violet rose connected to the energy and wisdom of a future heart that is about to create itself"

My early childhood vibrated abundance! My eyes could spark the magic within normal daily life. I felt strong and curious, playful and free when I was alone. In my family though, there was a kind of silence that moved through the rooms and around the dining room table...even the water was silent!

I learned over the years to enjoy the power and joy, the radiance and play, the inner abundance that came with me, in my alone time only. It felt like nobody was interested in sharing it with me anyway but in that, a gap was created. I missed real life happening around me, I missed connection, the integration of playfulness in my real life.

There was no play or fun and certainly not that much laughter as a child, I lived in the adults super serious world and in that space I lost connection to my own playfulness. It died, I lost my true self, the ease and the magic.

Years later, with my own children, I rediscovered that and reconnected with it. They were like rainbows for me, giving life back its colour and magic on a daily basis.

Play is so important, don't forget to reconnect with play if you've forgotten!

BREAKING THE HABIT OF NOT SPEAKING UP

"Overnight beautiful and exotic lime green flowers have been growing out of the soil.
In the morning they joyfully opened their extraordinary buds
and silently and lovingly, new energies introduced themselves
to the open hearts of the slowly awakening sleepers"

Sometimes I've felt like I've had something to say, some wisdom to add or knowledge to impart and I've silenced myself. My inner critic would smash my words to pieces and call me not worthy enough to speak out loud.

The last time I felt this way was at my son's wedding. It was nothing complicated actually, nothing difficult but I wasn't able to take the microphone and speak up. I wanted to let him and everyone else know how proud I felt about being his mother and how happy I was to welcome his wonderful wife into our family. This was two years ago and still, I feel the resentment and the stickiness of those unspoken words in my body.

But...that experience gave me the courage and permission to feel strong enough now to take my thoughts, put them into words and then give them a voice. It feels like a puzzle I'm now able to complete.

Darling, the world is missing something without your voice. Don't leave with unspoken words. Feel your thoughts, give them words and allow them your voice. Imagine them as the most beautiful flowers you get to create by yourself, let them bloom into the world.

CREATE CONNECTION ON YOUR TERMS

"That specific morning looked so different to the normal
that for some seconds, she was drawn to thinking
she was still stuck in an old dream.

A field of vibrating violet light opened up in front of her,
healing and repairing all old perceptions
that had been holding her back

New beliefs and patterns
beautifully started to plant themselves into
her inner fields of love and abundance"

Belonging is our human nature. We are created for connection and I think if this connection has gaps, then our existence is in danger. Permanent stress and the need to control, is what follows. I believe the lack of belonging is what influences our decisions in life, the partners we choose, the career we embark on and our own inner relationship with ourselves.

It took me half my life to realise that the feeling of not belonging anywhere, had led me to both inner and outer trouble. I hadn't chosen a job I loved and I didn't choose safe relationships, I'd been in constant inner tension.

At the age of forty-four, I made a decision to be more gentle with myself and really listen to my needs. I stopped responding to 'not belonging' and started understanding why my parents couldn't create that feeling of belonging and connectedness themselves. I also realised I was free to receive and connect to another source. This was the first time a deep connection and belonging to myself was established.

You my love don't have to wait that long. Be gentle with yourself and find your own special way of connecting.

DON'T UNDERESTIMATE THE POWER OF CELEBRATION

"The galactic conference was about to close,
when the energies finally agreed on opening the space between all times.
In that same instant, all human noise on earth stopped.
No more word was spoken, no more word could be heard.
This silence deeply resonated with the heart of mother earth.
A soft wind started to move the leaves of the trees and the waters of the rivers and oceans,
generating an intense, though subtle rhythm, reaching every human heart.
With that, waves and waves of golden yellow light
started to move gently around and between every human being,
repairing and healing past, present and future trauma and wounds.
Words started to become a different driver from that time onwards"

Looking back, I realise how powerful celebration is. Endings and beginnings need a moment of stillness and awareness to be received and integrated, to be witnessed. They are precious times of transition where magic happens without any effort. That's the beauty of celebration.

I always celebrated others for their achievements but I underestimated how much I was in need of being celebrated or being witnessed myself.

Instead of waiting for others to celebrate me, I started to integrate small celebrations for myself. Touching a precious stone, enjoying a beautiful flower, walking barefoot through water, creating something beautiful or delicious to eat.

I would listen to the sounds of the day and the sounds of my steps and really notice them. Those small celebrations helped to anchor the value I create in the world and to really appreciate myself. I do this every single day now.

So, celebrate yourself. Celebrate your life with small reachable things. Honour the place between the 'not yet' and 'no longer'.

Celebration gives us all the opportunity to connect to the timeless mystery of life, it's an important opportunity in integrating and cherishing all the lessons we've learned along the way.

INVITE THE HIDDEN PARTS OF YOU BACK HOME

In our neighbourhood there was an orphanage. From time to time, my father would threaten that if I continued to be such a difficult child, then there'd be no other option for my parents but to leave me there! That scared and shocked me.

Over the years, of course, I did my best to adapt to the demands of both my parents and my teachers. That meant swallowing my fears, my personality and my character. My life force in fact. It felt like taking those parts into the deepest darkness so nobody (including me) could ever reach them. I lived in survival mode.

As an adult, it took me a long time to travel back to those hidden parts, talk to them, inviting them to come back and connect again.

They came back in the form of poetry and they silently transmuted into the most beautiful diamonds I had ever seen! I started to write...

"Orphaned creation emerging from the depths of my being
I am calling you in with the silver lining of a soft February wind
that calms the inner storms of my unspoken words
and a curious inner child watching me, as I secretly start to own my voice"

So, if there are parts of you that have been hidden, start a sweet and tender conversation. Invite them in, over and over again. Create room and space so they can find themselves as part of you again, in an even more energetic and poetic way.

PERMISSION IS A GOLDEN LIGHT BETWEEN RESISTANCE AND DOUBT

There's a small line between doubt and resistance where I've always felt the need to choose between them. A pattern I repeated my whole life, I used resistance to not show up with my true power and voice. I doubted myself in order to hide my strength. I silenced myself constantly. Nobody in my environment would have to fear my power, my abundance, my creativity or my ease. It was a self-destroying pattern.

By the age of forty-four, I'd reached a point of self-sabotage that I could no longer manage. There were too many signs around me to ignore. Six female friends around my age and my mother died within six months – all unexpected. That was my turning point.

The truth wanted to come out and I surrendered. Giving myself permission to follow my heart rather than my brain, I took time out and went to the Ocean. I listened. Six weeks of listening and asking, without receiving any answer at all.

When I was about to leave, it hit me, all of a sudden. The waves showed me how life works, that it's all about rhythm, the coming and the going, the receiving and the letting go. It was like being flooded with a golden light of permission to be the woman that I truly was, to speak my truth and to show my full potential.

"Into the womb of sacredness, I immerse myself and gently receive and create from here"

If you feel doubt or resistance, sit in nature and let that golden light shine between both of them. Breathe and receive permission to grow and shine.

TRUST YOUR OWN VOICE

I find it hard to believe, how long I lived without ever trusting my heart. Every time there was a decision to be made, I made it with my mind, so disconnected was I from my intuition and heart. I can't blame my younger Self, it was simply a response to feeling unsafe.

I had a huge need to control (in order to feel safe), it felt like my true feelings were too dangerous to be listened to. With the help of a friend, I allowed myself to speak my truth for the very first time. It felt like an inner collapse of all false decisions and structures within me.

My heart immediately answered and what followed was an unstoppable need to move my body! I lost a lot of both body weight and story weight. I had a rebirth of my true Self. From one moment to the next, I felt safer and safer to be truthful and allow myself to feel whatever came up and my voice is still getting stronger and stronger as I continue to write poetry. I feel like my words are changing the narratives of women...

"She is the one who starts creating out of anticipation,
in a state of meticulously crafted presence,
allowing her borders and Mother Earths' borders to melt together
into one magic consciousness.
Opening deeply the emerging heart
and listening from here
to a greater story
and deeper wisdom
if you start listening with
your emerging heart to your own creation.
What would you want to listen to?
How blessed you are to wake up
to the beat of that golden beautiful heart?"

If you need a caring hand to hold yours while you speak a never before articulated truth, allow the universe to send it to you and your truth will be witnessed.

YOUR PAST IS NOT JUST YOUR PAST, IT'S YOUR ROOT SYSTEM

When I started exploring transgenerational trauma, it was the beginning of a completely different relationship with my mother. I asked her to tell me more about her childhood and her relationship with her parents.

We didn't end up in the deep conversation I'd hope for. Instead, she wrote the whole story down and sent it to me with all the documents she had from world war two and her family.

That opened another inner chamber of ancestral healing work. I deeply felt all her suffering and desperation. She was a little girl who lost her father in the war and waited for him her whole life. I'd unknowingly adopted that little girl my whole life too.

I knew I wouldn't be able to live freely unless I could let her go and allow my own roots to anchor into more nourishing soil. I knew that might also allow my Mother's roots to heal.

I wrote...

"My mothers hidden lakes secretly nested into magical landscapes
starting to connect silently with each other,
creating healing intimacy, indigo blue waters started
flooding the dry grounds of consciousness,
bringing back awareness to create new access to a deep belonging.
Opening up our future where presencing nature
enables the collective field to reconnect and restore itself,
it starts with reopening our internal land"

Unresolved ancestral trauma can be felt. If you feel it, imagine yourself as a root system, connected to a wider root system. Start to feel into the hidden and unseen, unheard parts of your ancestral lineage. Feel how welcomed you are and how your presence starts a deep healing, within yourself and your ancestors.

A film producer for twenty-five
years, her vision for words and
concepts has always been deeply
rooted in empathy and human
connection. Over the decades, she
has touched hearts with her words,
deepened relationships and found
self-love

Her soft but clear voice is loved by
so many. She felt she had
something of value to say in this
chapter and she was right.

Writing this was an opportunity
for her to dig deep and admit her
own authority with love, for the
benefit of other women.

@fluff_art

KATE 'FLUFF' THORNE

WHATEVER HAPPENS, GIVE THANKS

I chose to come here on planet earth. I chose my parents and all that came with them. I am, in actual fact, gratitude itself. When my beloved fell in love with someone else, I was absolutely devastated and shocked to the core. I cried for four months like never before, the grief and pain ripped me open as though a tsunami had hit my system!

I knew my response was way out of proportion to what had actually happened, all the grief and sorrow that I'd held over a very long time, seemed to take advantage of the situation and finally let go! Holy Cow! I thought the pain alone would kill me!

At the same time though, there was a deliciousness to it, I felt so alive, so present, so real, even sublime! Somewhere in me, I knew this was a blessing; gratitude sat sweetly in the background. I saw the innocence in me that got completely destroyed...seemingly.

I liken innocence with vulnerability, it's perhaps a more accurate word generally. I feel uncomfortable with the word vulnerability, it makes me feel powerless. However, 'innocence', can be touched, wounded and scarred but never destroyed entirely because it's pure.

So, while innocence remains, a maturity is gained by experience. I found this so beautiful to see and know in me. Whatever happens to me, I give thanks.

It also brings gratitude to all and allows for a greater understanding and compassion.

STAY ABSOLUTELY PRESENT

I had so much gratitude while looking after my parents. My mother had mild dementia, she confused her stories but otherwise was quite lucid. My father had Alzheimer's and his short-term memory rapidly decreased.

After my mother died, which happened quite suddenly, my father would ask where she was every day and often. After a few months, somehow, he got it but every time he remembered, it was as though it had just happened. They had been in love and inseparable for sixty-five years.

The teaching for me at this time was to stay more present than ever. The same questions from my father, required a loving response. I fondly called this my zen master training. As long as I remained present, he was fine. If I expressed the slightest impatience or annoyance, he would get confused and upset, as he had no idea he was repeating himself.

This whole time was such a privilege and an honour. Since then, I continue to be present effortlessly. Even when I'm disturbed, I'm present to that, everything and everyone is welcome to come and go in the oneness of silent awareness.

The most reliable and trustworthy place is Presence. It's still, alive, wise, loving, intelligent. From there the ability to respond is surprisingly easy, clear and honest. Less is more, less is more, less is more.

BE WITNESS TO YOUR BREATH

I witnessed three deaths in the space of eighteen months. These beings I love beyond words, my mother, my best four-legged friend and my father.

In death, there is a light that leaves the body, a spark of life, the breath. I witnessed it going in and out, until finally, they just stopped breathing in. It's very difficult to describe an energy departing, while a huge presence remains. It was deeply touching and humbling to understand the sacredness, the fragility, the vulnerability of the human breath.

Fall in love with breathing. I have experienced not breathing for some time, it has been like something is breathing me...Source...and Source doesn't even need to breathe!

Take great joy in the fact that you can take a deep breath in and exhale with such delight! How precious is this life! Contemplate the day you may stop breathing, it brings love back into life.

LOVE YOURSELF

I think everyone loves to talk about love! Great to remember in awkward social situations. As an adult, I had the experience of feeling the unique love my mother and father felt for me. I was so deeply touched by their blend of unconditional love, tenderness, innocence and the truth of it. I recognised in it, the godliness, the oneness, one heart, my heart, god's heart.

When the time came to love them as my children, I felt so happy and honoured to do so. My birth to their death, what a miracle. I see that as true reincarnation. I use the word God because once I realised God, then I understood it to be the best word for it but you could use Source or Love too, it means the same.

My greatest lover now, is me. When I tune in, I am the most alive, juicy and switched on 'divine yumminess' that I've ever known. Making love to myself in these moments, is orgasmic ecstasy and total union. I love to say 'I love you' to me and play love songs to myself, hearing the truth makes me happy and laugh out loud.

Sometimes I look in the mirror or see my reflection and just say 'I love you so much'. It feels great because it's true!

Love yourself, it's biggest work you'll ever do.

BE PRESENT...WITH YOU AND IN 'RELATION'SHIP

Take away the 'ship' from relationship and you'll find you have the opportunity to relate in the present moment. That means we can relate without the need for collecting ideas around what a relationship is, that inevitably builds a false identity, full of 'stuff' we don't need and actually it's constantly changing and in need of updating through conscious communication.

It means we can remain present without expectation, that we have the ability to respond and not react. That's far more exciting and harmonious, authentic, fresh and new, in every new 'now'. Share the freedom to be in the alive juicy flow of pure presence. It will turn you on! Think...

Less is more
Slow down
Pay attention
What's alive
Only now
Love is all

I've had the great fortune of awakening to this, our true nature and it's as mind blowing as it is simple. Just be quiet. Pretend you have no words, no vocabulary and no thoughts to be able to express anything. Like a baby, hmmmm, that's it, absolute perfection, nothing needs to be added, it's totally reliable and always available.

It is me. It is you. And it is we.

QUESTION EVERYTHING

I knew how much I didn't know but I had no idea how much I knew, that had to be let go of! I realised that the amount of conditioning and programming I'd accumulated from birth had been astonishing. My desire for freedom has required that I 'unlearn' all of it and start a fresh.

I like to be curious now, I like to question everything. I realised that any thoughts or ideas I had that didn't come from love were wrong thinking on my part. For me, if it's not loving, it's not it.

This has been so useful, knowing that any unkindness is a lie. Once I saw that, unloving thoughts lost their grip and started to give up. This kind of loving sees the bigger picture and understands that everyone and everything is connected without words.

I care deeply about others yet, through questioning everything, I remain carefree - as in 'being in the moment' and trusting that divine moments hold authentic, loving and intelligent responses.

Question everything.

THINGS I WISH I'D BEEN TOLD!

• You're not who you think you are, life is not what it seems and there is so much more to you than you realise.
• Who you are never dies, you can live as long as you like and your cells are reproducing themselves all the time
• What you believe is what will be, ask and you shall receive
• Love is the most powerful force in the Universe
• We are not separate, 'I' is you and 'you' is me, we are together and you are never alone
• You belong exactly where you are, always
• Intentions are powerful, make them, like prayers. Look for the win/win, life is always working for you... correction, with you!
• When making a difficult decision, choose the one that brings your mind the most peace
• Clear your energy daily with rituals that feel natural to you, take time to be alone in your own energy field, being unobserved has huge benefits!
• Cherish and nourish your sacred body, be sure about who you share it with, energies can get easily entangled and cause confusion just as easily as harmony
• If a man is able to truly be present with you, hear you and appreciate you, he is a healthy man.
• There are no mistakes!
• Shame is such an elusive feeling. I see it as the experience of turning away from what is true.

And lastly, you can change. You are the course of your life at any moment. I started as a firefighter, went on to be a film producer, then a psychotherapist followed by reiki master, body worker and energetic healer. In the last few years, I discovered an artist/painter in me and more recently I started writing.

I'm excited for the next chapter.

RETURN TO PEACE

'Do you believe this or that?' life says and I have to check and check again. Returning to peace always finds the right way. When I need to make a decision, I choose whichever gives me the most peace.

Return to peace.

Annie's husband Alistair has encouraged her to use her voice, believing in her so deeply. Her grandmothers encouraged her to sing and dance, telling her she could be whoever she wanted to be!

A strong woman to have in your corner, she believes that standing up for herself and knowing her boundaries is her life's work. She has 'fought like a lion' to protect those around her; most recently, she fought for her mother, ensuring her last years were dignified, respectful, faithful and loving.

Turning fear into fortitude, she stands on the ground her mother prepared for her, building her legacy into something as beautiful as she was.

@fearlessengagement

ANNIE SLOWGROVE-SCOTT

A POSITIVE FOCUS CONQUERS ALL

From being a little girl, I've had a sunshine outlook. I love to dance and sing, get dressed up and go play in the mud (still do that too).

I believe that life is full of interesting, marvellous, strange and fascinating things. And then, stuff happens. In my early twenties, as a hotel manager, I was on my feet a lot.

Walking became painful and so steroids were prescribed...along with a wheelchair!

Within months, I was diagnosed with rheumatoid arthritis. They said I should give up work and accept that life would be difficult now. I understood the words but every part of me shouted 'That's not me!'.

Terrified but balancing fear with a positive (humorous) outlook that I would not be beaten, I greedily read everything I could on my condition. I think the more you know about something, the more you can understand its reason for being, work with the symptoms and beat it.

I discovered research on the link between nutrition and rheumatoid arthritis. So I started excluding foods, experimenting, liquidising veggies and drinking bottled water.

I reintroduced foods slowly, some put my progress back weeks! But my confidence grew. I was out of the wheelchair on crutches (freedom) within a year and two years later was dancing and gardening with my Grandad!

Always begin with mindset! Acknowledge your fears, don't ignore them, invite them in.

Trust and believe in your deep innate courage as a human to be more, do more and achieve more.

You have a choice.

Make your own decisions, don't blindly trust others. It's your life, you choose!

CHOOSE THE WORDS AND THE MOVIE WILL MAKE ITSELF!

I have a reputation for being calm in any storm. And I like being calm but I don't always feel it. One morning, a friend sent me a link to a spiritual weekend 'You're going with me!' she said.

Two months later, I'm sitting in a circle with eight lovely people, candles and incense when I began to feel oddly alone. Asked why we'd attended, I said 'I'm here to reconnect with Annie'.

Out of the mouth of our spiritual teacher came the words "Can I give you what I feel Annie, when I look at you?...NUMB!'

Tears fell, the room stood still and I was transported to age nine in a field in a tent. I lost my breath totally. I felt like I was swimming on the ceiling looking down on myself. I didn't know that the situation I was recalling was even a thing, I'd forgotten or rather papered over it, creating a numbness I learned to live with and coated as calm.

I was assaulted. Oh the shame I'd lived with suddenly crushed me. I'd created numbness to protect myself. I feel I've moved past this trauma stronger and better now. I've found peace, I have no horrible memory but the story we tell ourselves becomes the life we live. I took the word NUMB and created acronyms...

Day 1: Nowhere for Us to have Moments to Breathe
Day 3: Nuances of Understanding with Moments of Bliss
Day 5: Never Underestimate My Brilliance
Day 7: Never-ending Unique Moments of Brilliance

And finally: New Understandings Make me Bolder!

Words change worlds, your inner world is a beautiful landscape of experience, all laced with its own language. Choose the words and the movie will make itself!

GIVE YOURSELF PERMISSION

I was taught that good girls were seen and not heard. Very good little girls were seen, not heard and did what they were told too! I followed 'life' rules, I learned to fit in and be who others wanted me to be and I did it well! The problem with living through the lens of rules though, is that you seek approval from others, from what you wear or the hairstyle you have, you may think you're making your own choices (as I did) but it's the rule choosing – not you!

In my forties, something snapped. I didn't want to fit in anymore. I resigned from my job, took a leap of faith and joined the self-employed. So many voices told me not to, they thought I should stay in the safe lane. Fed up with others telling me I was too much, too loud, too quiet or too anything, I did what I wanted.

Don't waste your time trying to fit in. We somehow believe it brings connection and belonging but it's only you, you need to connect with. You are enough as you are, stop chasing shadows; sit quiet and feel YOU.

The most important relationship you will ever have, is the one you have with yourself. Bring your whole self wherever you go, that's how you'll move through the world confident, grounded and comfortable in your own skin, with an understanding of who you are and what you're about.

Give yourself permission to be who you really are.

LET THE WORDS FALL OUT

One day at Sunday breakfast, with no appetite and my heart pounding in my ears, I heard myself say "Can we talk about us?". The words just fell out, almost like they'd been given life. The separation conversation continued by starting somewhere. Anywhere.

I began to speak. To say what I wanted and needed. We are constantly invited to be who we are in conversation, to share our real words, our unfiltered essence – if we take the invitation by the hand.

And if you do and can speak of your feelings, needs, boundaries and desires, your authenticity is evident to all. It's taken me years to learn how to communicate this way.

Somewhere beneath the layers of people-pleasing, white lies and insecurity I carried, I knew there was a bold, confident, self-actualised woman. I wanted, more than anything, to become her. On the journey to becoming that woman, I learned that authentic communication is like working a muscle: hard at first but easier with exercise.

Warm up your voice by letting the words fall out and give life to the fantastic, confident, genuinely wonderful human being you are, one conversation at a time. It could well be imperfect and messy at first, that, in itself, is wonderfully bold and liberating.

Through the intention of love, let your words fall out as you hold tight to the essence of you and everything will work out.

LETTING GO OF PERFECTION

I'd like to say I am a reformed perfectionist but I'm a work in progress. I've been an obsessive perfectionist in the past, losing nights of sleep over the smallest of mistakes which led to anxiety and body issues.

Years ago, I pitched for a new piece of work that would change our lives. I spent days and nights writing slides and practicing my lines. The presentation was beautiful, it looked amazing, pictures looked fabulous on the big screen, my team and I practised together, we were all word perfect.

The morning of the pitch, I decided the pictures weren't good enough and made the team redo over half the presentation!

When the time came, we were indeed word perfect. Two days later though I received the call. We didn't win the work. "Thank you to your team Annie, they were really great, relaxed and funny too but, we won't be inviting you back...you were too polished Annie, we didn't feel that we got the real you in the room", I was ashamed and devastated! I decided in that moment to change.

Being perfect was instilled in me so it has been no easy journey. My main trait back then, was to make something LOOK perfect but what's often missing then, is meaning. Nowadays I try to shift my focus on 'finding meaning'. If something brings joy and purpose, then it doesn't matter if it's not done perfectly.

'Meaning over perfection' is now on a large canvass in my office as a reminder! Here's to being enough, not perfect but enough!

NEVER LET SOME ELSE'S BEHAVIOUR DOMINATE YOURS

I had butterflies! My first time allowed out with a boy, on a bus to the flicks. I remembered my Mams words, in that tone, 'Be back by 10pm. Don't be late'.

Being even one minute late meant walking into hysterics, screaming, crying and a bloody good telling off. That night...the bus was late. As I walked through the gate, I heard her wailing. Mam was being comforted by Grandma, Grandad, Aunties, Uncles, even my cousins! And... the police had been called. I felt the fear and held back the tears, again!

I was six minutes late! To my Mam that meant I'd been raped and murdered. Her fear, even today, is uncontrollable, irrational and terrifying.

By my twenties, I did as I was told, keeping Mam's world in harmony. By thirty, I'd divorced and moved counties to escape her gaze but fast forward to forty-three, she fulfilled her dream and moved 600 miles to be closer to me!

By forty, I'd divorced and moved counties to get away from her gaze but fast forward to fifty-three and they moved over 600 miles to be closer to me! Fuck...what now?

After divorce number two, near bankruptcy, I moved counties again. I can and must make the choice that's right for me. I knew I had to break her harmony or my own heart!

I stopped doing as I was told, listened to my own voice and found happiness. I've set boundaries around my needs, my opinions and my life. Mam's now eighty-two and hasn't changed. But I have!

You never have to behave as others demand, you'll lose your spark as I did and no-one has the right to take that away! Know your boundaries and guard them like a lion!

FOOTNOTE:

During writing this, my Mam passed away. Her death has impacted me as any death does; sadness and loss play their tune in our hearts. But it's given me an insight into fear. My Mam feared life itself and her actions towards me were really towards herself. She was trying to protect herself. She was doing her best, I know. But she lost her spark too, because fear was the only emotion she knew how to be with. Let go of fear; if you don't, it will rob you of life, your life. Get up, get busy, get out there and be YOU! Stop waiting. Grab life. It won't come unless it's invited.

THE MOST IMPORTANT RELATIONSHIP IS THE ONE WITH YOURSELF

Sitting beside my Mammy's hospital bed, holding her hand and stroking her hair, I deeply felt love for her, more than I can ever remember. I wasn't sad, I was shocked. I felt an inner strength and a profound love and commitment I'd never experienced. I began to explore these new feelings. Until now, I'd managed my relationship with my Mam from a distance. I realised that managing relationships separated me from others and significantly, from myself.

I wanted to feel, express and enjoy being in the moment and hold tight to her joyful smile and this new feeling of powerful love and commitment. I knew deep down I needed to strengthen my relationship with myself! Starting with some basics.

I tried to figure out what I wanted; I knew no-one could take that away once I knew. I wanted to practice love. I knew I could only experience the true beauty of love once I understood it and developed a loving relationship with myself. And I sought to find my wisdom...that combination of knowledge and character.

I had no idea in my sixties, that my Mam would gift me one of the greatest lessons of my life. It was like in that hospital room, I was reborn with a renewed life force, that 'love lies at the seat of powerful commitment'. And from there, a relationship with myself sprang.

Your relationship with yourself is significant, it's the foundation for all your relationships. If you have a strong, stable relationship with yourself, you can be strong and stable in your other relationships. You'll be in the best place to love and help them grow, while their love helps you grow.

TRUST YOURSELF, IF YOU DON'T - HOW CAN OTHERS?

'How do you trust yourself?' I asked at a training event. I was given answers like: knowing what your values are, doing what you say you're going to do, showing up for others, standing up for what you think is fair and right...

That last one, somehow, floated into my head and wouldn't shift. I'm the 5ft 1" woman who makes youngsters take their feet of the seat on trains. I face down anyone who's unkind or bullying another. I was even a bouncer in my own hotel and taught others how to stand their ground! I know how to stand up for what's right but the feeling that I didn't trust myself kept coming back.

One night at dinner, as the conversation became energetic, people disagreeing with one another, I began holding back my thoughts. Feeling hot and uncomfortable, I fell silent. I went home, straight to bed, buried my head in my pillow and sobbed.

I finally fell asleep, opening my eyes to songbirds and sunshine. As I sat in the conservatory at five o'clock in the morning, drinking tea in my favourite cup, I heard a little voice say 'No-one is judging you now Annie. It's okay to be yourself. Trust in yourself. You are enough'.

I realised I'd learned to be the person others wanted. I was afraid of being judged and literally in that moment, my confidence came through and I said to myself in a strong voice 'I am a strong, funny, intelligent, kind and slightly wacky woman. I can do and handle anything but only if I trust in myself! I'm still work in progress but I'm better than ever.

Trust yourself

Morna's inspiration to speak up came from the indomitable Maya Angelou, she was so inspired by her fearless, passionate and rebellious words. Encouraged by friends and family, the importance of using her voice came later in life; she was a great advocate for others but seldom for herself.

"Self-love," she declares now, "alongside a wise woman's voice, is indeed a revolution!"

"Not so long ago," she continues, "women couldn't vote, let alone impart advice without being burnt at the stake. So, what a privilege it is to be able to have a voice and write as part of this incredible book, empowering both the writer and reader.

@mjmitchell_writer

MORNA MILTON-WEBBER

IF YOU'VE BEEN ADOPTED, SEEK OUT YOUR SOUL TRIBE

Feelings of abandonment and rejection never seem far away from those of us who were given up for adoption. For me, it's been a pain that runs so deep, it's actually visceral. An ache that has coursed through my veins, I have constantly sought deliverance from the torment.

The mother wound is forever open for me, salved at times but never fully healed. I haven't found anything that has made up for the loss of a mother and the feelings attached to my birth experience are powerful.

But to live a full and authentic life, I had to make sense of it all. I had to treat my brokenness with the utmost kindness.

Validation came from finding out that others were experiencing the same feelings of hopelessness. I had my OMG moment reading Nancy Verrier's 'Primal Wound', it discussed the wound that results when a child is separated from his/her mother and the subsequent trauma that ensues. I had to finally admit that I was struggling with feelings of being unlovable, unworthy, empty and angry.

My saving grace came in various forms. Counselling was important (I found someone who specialised in adoption), I read and explore others experiences (it really did help) and I met up with other kindred spirits... adoptees who could completely relate to me.

Those were my veritable lifeline. Trust me! There is nothing more potent and healing than finding your soul tribe, those who truly see you, empathise, understand and 'get' you.

BE PROUD OF THE CHOICES YOU MADE WHEN YOU DIDN'T KNOW ANY BETTER

I have been in a crazy stomach growling, heart howling relationship with food for most of my life. I'm a seasoned emotional eater.

A cavernous feeling of emptiness engulfed me when, at five years old, I found myself desperately trying to survive the harsh, cold environs of a strict boarding school. Trying to find a way to fill an emotional void, starved of affection and love, I found solace and comfort in food. Eating soon became my way of soothing my distress, sadness, isolation and fear plus it was a way to suppress pain and a variety of negative emotions.

As a child, I had no understanding of coping mechanisms or the psychology of it all. I just did what I had to, to survive the trauma and numb the agony. This was my way of existing through childhood, adolescence and into maturity.

Whilst I've gone through a lifetime on the overeating cycle 'eat - self comfort - guilt - weight gain - poor self-image - upset – eat', I am, believe it or not, genuinely proud of myself.

Throughout the years, many other opportunities to disconnect presented themselves...drugs, alcohol and I chose perhaps the least destructive. I continue to try to stop walking away from myself, to tackle my comfort eating, to do inner child work and sit with my flawed humanity - despite it being uncomfortable, challenging and frightening. I'm complicated, intricate, complex, exquisitely unique but I am me. And I honour that.

FIND YOURSELF

Against all the rules and regulations, I took my son out of primary school for two years and we travelled the length and breadth of India and South East Asia in a vintage 1935 Rolls Royce with no power steering or power assisted brakes!

We journeyed the coconut palm clad shores of Kerala, drove the deserts of Rajasthan, watched the sunrise above Mount Everest and set again over Annapurna, Nepal. We visited a leper colony in Nagpur and stood in silence at the stupa of skulls at Pol Pot's Phnom Penh killing fields in Cambodia. We walked the bridge over the River Kwai at Kanchanaburi in memory of the 16,000 allied prisoners of war who died, swam in the mighty Mekong river and explored the lost kingdom of Angkor Wat.

All these experiences allowed us to learn and talk about the travesties of war, discuss the diversity of cultures around the world, the legacies left by corrupt and despotic leaders, witness the effects of climate change, understand first-hand what it's like to live with disability, disease and abject poverty. Those adventures taught my son so much more than he could ever have learnt from text books and I believe he's a much more humbled, grounded and resilient young man now because of our wanderlust.

Education comes in many forms and travel is an extraordinary teacher. Perhaps the most valuable thing we learnt together from our expeditions, was gratitude. As a family, we're thankful for all the many opportunities we have and we appreciate the things we used to take for granted, like a roof over our heads, food, clean water, education, our freedom and feeling safe.

Please, don't let fear of the unknown stop you living your best life. Venture outside your comfort zone to find yourself. I did. It not only opened my eyes but also my heart. I have a much deeper respect for this incredible planet we are blessed to live on and I'm better able to think beyond my own challenges and realise the adversities faced by others.

YOU ARE NOT YOUR HAIR!

Much as I don't like to admit it, I have felt defined as a woman by my looks and by my hair, so when I started to lose my hair, it often had me in tears, accompanied by days when I couldn't leave the house. Hair loss affects millions of women around the world, somehow, it's accepted in men but not women and it's where the shame and hatred for how I looked has stemmed from.

Glancing in the mirror and catching sight of my scalp shining through and the horror of discovering bald patches was upsetting, especially when every magazine and social media picture glorifies women with thick, healthy flowing locks.

I learned to embrace and accept my situation though, slowly understanding that - I am not my hair, my looks or my body. I am still a worthy wonderful woman whether I have hair or not. I needed to look inside and do some soul searching, to look deeper than the superficial nonsense made up by corporations who still conspire to sell me a fantasy world making me feel inadequate and worthless.

Changing my mindset and the false marketing narrative was key for me. My hair loss now represents my triumphs from the health battles I have had to fight. When I look in the mirror now, I'm proud of how I have survived. I appreciate that I'm wonderfully incomparable and beautiful in my own way.

A LETTER TO THE WOMAN WHO THINKS SHE'S UNLOVABLE

I read somewhere that "You are not unlovable because someone important to you, didn't know how to love you". What a powerful statement!

Often the people I have looked to for love, acceptance or attention were too broken themselves to give me the affection, tenderness and warmth that I so yearned.

That didn't make the situation acceptable and it most certainly didn't excuse their behaviour but by acknowledging someone else's pain, it allowed me to see things from a different perspective. Sadly, the 'important' people in my life simply didn't know how to heal their own trauma and effectively handed it to me. I don't think I'm alone. I believe many of us have had to carry a load that wasn't ours to bear.

Recognising that has been incredibly difficult, yet, so vitally imperative for me because in doing so (and against all I had been told or shown), I found that I always HAD been lovable - it just took me a long time to recognise the truth. I had been living their lie with such credibility!

Here's to lessons learned, to always being open to changing the perspective, to self-love, healing and acceptance. I honour myself and give much respect to all the other chain breakers in this world, to those of us who do the authentic, challenging, messy work of healing.

Acknowledging the brokenness and pain of others, allowed me to fight my way out of the dark shadows of self-loathing and doubt, maybe it will help you too.

Let's celebrate and be proud - an invisible army of unstoppable, brave, strong soul sister warriors doing the work and loving ourselves, so we can love others in the true sense.

NEVER TAKE THE GIFT OF LIFE FOR GRANTED

I sat vigil at my son's bedside in hospital, he couldn't breathe and his chest was concave. I'd cradled him in the ambulance, wrapping him in the arms of mother's love.

A hospital environment is filled with all manner of obnoxious odours...but my fear...was the most potent of all. I was terrified at the sight of four white coats standing at the bottom of his bed. They were asking for permission to do an emergency tracheotomy. It was all very surreal, I remember my desperate need to pray, to plead with the Universe, every God, deity, Source or power that be, to spare the life of my boy.

One last spray of steroid down the throat before theatre and suddenly, a miracle. He gasped a huge gulp of air and began breathing. Slowly but surely, oxygen reaching his lungs.

I came close to losing my son that day. The tough lesson is the stark reality of the fragility of life, this gift of existence each of us is given at birth. There isn't a day goes by that I'm not grateful to see him grow into the wonderful young man he is today. I am truly blessed.

YOU CAN DO THIS!

Climbing out of a dark place takes steely determination and grit. But you can do this! For me, there came a time amidst the chaos and turmoil of my marriage, when I instinctively knew the time was right.

I remember the pivotal moment when I stopped being madly in love and replaced 'staying together' with an exit strategy that was forming in the recess of my frazzled and exhausted brain.

The uncertainty and fear set in. What will I do? How will I cope? Will there be enough money? Why is this happening? Where will I go? My self-doubt was as crippling as the crumbling marriage I had to leave. The unknown was terrifying.

I had to make friends with courage and embrace self-love and respect because it wasn't easy to make such a monumental life change, especially when I was hanging on emotionally by just a thread.

My words to you are 'don't give up on yourself - remember your worth should never be determined by outside forces'.

Go find yourself again, remember the wonderful human being you are and fall back in love with you. Chase your dreams and put yourself first.

Don't ever settle for putting up with a situation because you're too scared to leave. You are worth so much more than that. Trust that you are always enough just as you are.

USE YOUR VOICE

It took a massive four inch cut to my throat, a partial thyroidectomy and the removal of a cancerous tumour to make me realise the value of my voice.

My throat has always been my weak point. If I got a cold, it would invariably end up as pharyngitis, tonsillitis, strep throat...I would simply lose my voice. In reality I never used my voice properly because I didn't feel I had anything important to say!

When I was emotionally upset, my throat felt constricted. I'd try to vocalise my feelings and feel shut down. Choked. Deep down, I knew it was a lack of self-worth, not feeling worthy of being heard. When my surgeon warned that the surgery might affect my voice (being so close to my vocal chords) and that I might sound different or even lose my voice completely, I was shocked. I couldn't imagine not being able to talk...yet, I'd lived in self-inflicted silence when I'd had the ability to speak all along!

In that moment, I recognised that whilst situations and people had contributed to me not using my voice, I'd always had power to change it, I just hadn't seen it.

I vowed from that moment that I would awaken! I'd find my voice and heal from a lifetime of 'not feeling good enough'. And I have. Everyone should know they can use their voice.

There are two women who have
inspired Kath to find her voice:
her wonderful, warm and funny
mum, Rae and her friend and
'age-inspiration' - elder of this book,
Kate Peace.

She is a daughter, a sister, a mother
and grandmother to a delicious two-
year-old granddaughter, already an
explorer, scientist, artist and dancer!

She was inspired to use her voice in
this book specifically because it
supports children who aren't having
the childhood they deserve.
 However, she goes on to say that
"Sometimes, it's not spoken words
that are needed, it's an excruciatingly
carefully crafted compassionate text
or a five-breath-long hug".

KATH MORGAN-THOMPSON

SAVE YOURSELF, YOU CAN

When I was sixteen living away at sixth form college, I felt very sad and low. It was cold, raining and 1979, as I phoned my mum from the red telephone box, where you needed the right change and your coins were always on the verge of running out.

Heralded by the urgency of 'the pips' (beeping sounds that always seem to curtail any phone box conversation, good or bad), Mum told me that hundreds of girls would be grateful to be in my shoes and to have the opportunity I had. She more or less said 'pull up your sloppy socks and get on with it!'.

I had hoped she would weave some magic motherly words of comfort and that she could lift me into a warm light place of 'it's going to be alright'. I wanted her to save me from the leaden dark heart that my age and hormones had given me to drag around. Save me!

I didn't know at that time that she needed a warm light much more than me. We don't notice other people's burdens when we're struggling with our own. I found out later that she had a big mountain of shite on her plate that day. But, as the pips went, I had a realisation. She'd done me a massive favour. I realised that no-one can 'save' me from my own life. People can give us a leg up the ladder sure, someone can shine a light on the more treacherous slippery parts of our path or drag us into a lifeboat but survival must come from inside us...alone. You save yourself.

And if it seems impossible, start in one tiny corner, just one little thing, even if it's the next few breaths or putting on the kettle or splashing your face with cold water. Save yourself this time and then the next time and you'll get a taste for it.

LEAVE THE COBWEBS AND DUST!

Somebody I knew once died from falling downstairs carrying a hoover...if that doesn't make you consider giving up housework, I don't know what will!

It's probably a good idea to keep the bathroom and food prep areas hygienic (if you're lucky, they're not in the same room) but if you're not asthmatic, I strongly advocate loosening up about cobwebs and dust, just a bit.

Even Miss Haversham from Great Expectations survived a prolonged period without flicking a duster around and Quentin Crisp once said the dust doesn't deepen after four years! My mum is eighty-five years old and lives in the countryside in Wales. She has macular degeneration in one eye and gets injections for it every six weeks. She has one of the best excuses for literally turning a nearly blind eye to the arachnids' architecture.

She's been cleaning her house with an extendable feather duster for years and by the time she's got round the living room, the beasties are throwing up new constructions where she started, you can almost hear them singing while they're spinning.

Of course, do it if it makes you feel good but my advice is feel free to leave it! And if anyone comes round to your house tutting at your lacey crevices, don't open the biscuit tin and show them the damn door!

RETAIN 'YOU' IN A LONG-TERM PARTNERSHIP

I've been married nearly thirty-nine years, that's a long time. Being in a marriage long term requires not only patience and humour but it also requires us to keep our own personal twinkle.

Good friends are essential. I've taken my soul to the harbour of their company where I can throw myself into listening to them and they to me. I've moved my arse! Yoga, dance, walking...have boosted my resilience and recharged my 'joy for life' battery.

I've retained my spark by creating, by dropping my energies into new ideas. I count the blessings in life and find myself drawn to those who are struggling, to be useful to them. I've studied too...the wisdoms, the books, Ted Talks, podcasts and I've learned to pray for guidance.

Find ways to keep YOU afloat, not only your relationship. Keep yourself alive and thriving through the stormier times and you'll sail back into the sunshine when the clouds clear!

YOU'RE STRONGER THAN YOU THINK

I've often thought about life being like a gym. I have stretched my imagination here, having avoided all gyms apart from the smelly one at school but bear with me. In the gym, you lift weights. Eventually, the weights no longer feel as hard to lift, so you lift heavier ones. The new weights are hard to lift and you get all sweaty again but, of course, you're training your muscles to be stronger. Life has borrowed that concept I feel.

'Here you are!' life says, 'Stick this on your shoulders!'. I've thought it would break me, almost impossible to hold at first but as I've stuck with it, it all became easier. Sometimes life gives you a back breaking weight and it feels like you can't budge it! But keep your form, enlist a bit of assistance from others and you'll lift it.

What I'm trying to get at here, with this ridiculous and somewhat torturous metaphor, is that, the heavy bits of life can be helpful if you think of them as training.

Strength does not develop in the changing room; it happens in the gym. Strength without flexibility is stiffness and flexibility without strength is floppiness. No-one wants floppy.

Pay close attention to our body and mind, then load, stretch and work wisely. Develop resilience, pull on your metaphorical Lycra thong leotard and get stuck into life!

TRY YOGA

I started going to yoga a bit reluctantly to be honest. A friend was training to be a teacher and needed bums on mats. I am of the pre-video/DVD generation that did Jane Fonda 'go for the burn!' workouts from an actual LP! So I was somewhat cynical about this hippy dippy yoga palaver. No sweat? No suffering? Just breathing, stretching and relaxing.

Slowly, after a few months of regular practice, I noticed I was getting less moody and bitchy, more relaxed and comfy in my own skin, more peaceful in my heart and mind. I needed to study this yoga business and perhaps pass on the wisdoms! Ashleigh Brilliant the aphorist wrote 'I may not be totally perfect but parts of me are excellent'. At sixty, it's now my motto and one that my yoga students can relate to as well.

I've been teaching yoga for about sixteen years now. My students don't want to stand on their heads or put their feet behind their ears, instead they want peace and joy, they want fun. They want a break from being a grown-up, from doing tough life stuff like coping, caring and grieving.

Yoga is a lovely thing, it doesn't cost the earth and you don't need fancy gear. You don't need to be fit, young, bendy or trendy. Breathing is the only thing that's mandatory.

My aim is to get people who consider themselves not yoga-y to try it and want to bring their best friend next week. I'm hoping to plant a little yoga seed in the back of your mind. One day you will see a yoga poster in the chip shop and maybe you'll give it a go, even if, like me, you're a bit of a cynic.

LOVE THE LABELS YOU GIVE YOURSELF

I haven't really known who I am until recently. I mean who I REALLY am. I've had loads of labels...mother, granny, daughter, wife, sister, cleaner.

I used to hate the labels in my clothes, feeling judged by my dress size - don't look at my bum! Now I rather like the labels that society says I shouldn't have 'at my age' – comedian, performance artist and stripper! I really like those ones.

I've only acquired these in the last decade. It was like, my ovaries' ability to produce hormones decreased at exactly the same time that my urge to show off increased!

I've started calling myself a 'sexygenarian' - which is ironic because I have no libido and it's too late to juice back up with HRT if I don't fancy a heart attack or stroke. According to a male GP!

You're still thinking about the stripper bit aren't you? I shall explain. At the age of fifty-two, I was dragged to a charity burlesque show. My jaw hit my knees. Beautiful, magnificent, gorgeous creatures taking their clothes off with swagger and sass and style. Not one an airbrushed Barbie doll of a thing.

Real women, stretch marks, bellies and sensational cellulite topped off with sequins and sparkle. I went home that night and revolutionised my relationship with my bum. I did a course with Lily Labelle in a darts room in Harrogate, where I devised an alter ego middle-aged cleaning lady and I've been performing ever since.

I don't get my tits out by the way, the breastfeeding, gravity and trampolining have left them ravaged. But my question to you is 'Who are you really?'.

BE PATIENT WITH YOURSELF, YOU CAN HEAL AND OVERCOME ANYTHING

'Live in the moment!' they say. In the last year of my fifties, I did not want to live in the moment, I didn't actually want to see the year out.

I'd developed a rapidly destructive, inflammatory sort of mysterious arthritis. It felt like my skeleton was savagely rotting on the inside...both hips, right knee, neck and thumbs.

I like to think that inside us, we have a spark of life, a pilot light of joy and hope but mine was wavering and shrinking with each day. The orthopaedic surgeon said my condition was unusual but I wasn't unique. Rude! (We all want to be special!).

He replaced my hips and knee in the end, love that man! Recovery was hard physically and psychologically but I used all my yoga techniques of breathing, relaxation, meditation and visualisation. (The Yoga Nidra recording of Swami Pragyamurti was my loyal companion on long, painful pre and post op nights).

I drew on these powers and so can you. Find what protects and nurtures your pilot light and feed it regularly. I clung to my quivering pilot light flame and, with each operation, it grew just a tiny bit.

Be patient with your healing process. Sometimes you need to just get through the moment and not think about the next. Feed the flame, in whatever way makes sense to you, keep your hope alive and the trust the joy will return, it will!

FIND THE FUNNY AND RIDICULOUS...IT'S ALWAYS THERE

I have a super-power! I always find the humour in every situation however bleak. I find if you hit the right comic note in either word, expression or attitude, light floods down from above and a connection is made between you and your comedic co-conspirator!

A spark of joy burns away some of the pain of the moment. They say, humour is the crack that lets the light in.

I like to see the 'crack' in someone's face too...they break into a smile, teeth flash, eyes twinkle, wrinkles crinkle and dopamine squirts! Moods shift, coping mechanisms are brought back online. You, my love, are not alone.

I've self-regulated by doing this...apart from some hormonal glitches in my teens and one godawful contraceptive pill which I named 'psycho-gynon', I consider myself very blessed that I've found the ridiculous, as my base setting.

Life splats out manure as well as sunshine and we're ALL in the firing line at some point! But... there's always a funny or ridiculous. It might feel elusive but even the process of looking for it, does as much as the finding of it!

It has been Mikel heart's desire to be
surrounded by wise women, to sit in
their presence and learn from their
wisdom. Now, she finds herself
doing exactly that as she shares her
own voice and wisdom in her second
collaborative book, connecting with
women around the globe.

She credits Lynette Allen as being
one of many women who have
inspired her to use her voice—a voice
that is now more potent than ever.

As a courageous leader, a devoted
medicine facilitator and coach,
Mikel uses her voice and wise words
daily to inspire, encourage and heal
not only herself but those who bring
themselves to her door too.

@mikelannhall

MIKEL ANN HALL

A MOTHER'S LOVE CAN BE FOUND IN UNEXPECTED PLACES

I never experienced the depths of a mother's love until I was in my fifties. It came from a Vietnamese woman. I'd been living in Vietnam with a family, a mother, father and two girls.

One night I was awakened by a light passing through my room. There was an intruder in the house. I laid still, pretending to be asleep. Eventually the light moved on. The next morning, I told the family, through my charades and the little bit of English I'd taught the youngest girl, what had happened.

Distraught, the father left and returned with CCTV cameras. Later that evening, I noticed a light in the front room still on. It was Mom. Her sleeping mat lay just behind the front door, a mosquito net strung over it.

She turned at the sound of my footsteps. As I looked at her lying on the floor, she knew what I was thinking and silently nodded yes. I crouched down, as a tear ran down my cheek, realising she was going to sleep between the front door and my room to protect me. As we reached for each other, I saw pure love in her eyes, looking into mine. In that one embrace, I truly felt a mother's love for the very first time.

I'd never experienced such a moment with my own mother. I do fondly remember a time when my mother's eyes welled up with tears as she looked at me taking in all that I had become and in that moment, I knew she was proud of me.

In her own ways, my mother really did love me. I just hadn't recognised it. She taught me to love, to nurture, protect and keep safe the little girl within me. This gift in itself, is love. I see that now, knowing love can be expressed in many different ways and doesn't always look the way we imagine it would.

WE CAN DO ALL THINGS THROUGH FAITH

I had closed my eyes to allow the depth of the impact to settle. Seconds before, I'd sailed through the air, crashing onto asphalt; I'd just 'taken a door', (when a driver opens their car door without looking properly and causes a cyclist to crash!).

I opened them to a sea of cycling shoes and bare feet. The feet had voices. I focused on the one that said, "I'm a doctor". "Can you stand?" he asked. "I don't know" I said. I felt shoulders come underneath my arms as I was supported in standing and immediately collapsed. A siren wailed in the distance. I realised it was for me. As I was loaded into the back of the ambulance, I noticed a tattoo on the inside of the EMT's arm, 'Be present' it said. I laughed, my angels were with me.

I felt God's presence in the emergency room as the doctor told me I was out! I wouldn't be racing. I felt calm and supported as he explained what had happened to my body and how they were going to repair it.

A few weeks after surgery, tears flooded down my cheeks as my physical therapist encouraged me to relearn how to step off a curb! I sobbed. How had I gotten here? I was standing on a curb afraid and not knowing how to step down, when I should have been half way around the world competing in my second Ironman!

As the tears fell, I felt God compassionately listening and allowing me to speak all my woes. He dried my tears as I looked up into the heavens and said, "Okay, I'm ready. Help me". With a determined focus and courage, knowing I could do all things through Him, one foot, then the other, I stepped down. I squealed in delight beaming with joy as I stepped up again. I'd done it!

As my body slowly healed, I was haunted by the sound of my bike hitting the door. I prayed and asked God to take the sound away and He did. I never heard it again!

God knows the tears and the pain in our hearts. Be strong and courageous. Do not be afraid for He has glorious plans to prosper you, not harm you. He promises strength for the days, comfort for the tears and light for the way.

DREAMS REALLY DO COME TRUE

Once upon a time there was a little girl who wanted to be a mermaid and grow up to be just like her grandmother. Travelling to distant lands, exploring faraway places, swimming in the depths of the world's deep blue seas and living a life in awe!

She spent hours sitting at the feet of her grandmother, eagerly listening to the wizened woman speak of her tall tales and adventures. "Grandmother, one day when I grow up, I wanna be just like you!"

As she grew up, she always reflected fondly upon these musings. In college, she learned about visualisation. Olympic athletes, even astronauts were trained in visualisation and had been doing it for years. So she began.

Inspired by a man she met who'd climbed Mount Everest, she visualised trekking to Base Camp with him... and she did. A year later, to celebrate her fiftieth birthday, she visualised doing an Ironman and finishing in less than fifteen hours...and she did, crossing the finish line in 14:57.

She learned that not only seeing the desired result but using all her senses to feel it, were key. Many years later, post-surgery, swept away by grief at not being able to walk and on the brink of giving up, she remembered. If I can feel it and see it, I can achieve it. Teaching herself to walk again wasn't always easy, yet she persevered... and she did.

She walked down to the sea and felt the warmth of the soft white sand between her toes, the water tickling her feet and for the very first time in a long time, she smiled.

She did grow up to be just like her grandmother and is enjoying a life of travelling to distant lands, exploring faraway places, swimming in the depths of the world's deep blue seas and living in awe!

GO WITH THE FLOW

My sailor's mouth went off, as I spewed out the most colourful and vehement profanities I knew. I'd just been hit by an oncoming car's side mirror, as the driver careened, too fast (in my opinion) down a narrow road towards me. As I rubbed my shoulder, I was aware of the anger and tension within. I'd never experienced road rage before driving a motorbike in Asia! I felt reactive, my vision narrowed and my heart was racing.

I learned to drive in the west, with rules. Asia is different. There's a flow within the chaos of their roads. 'Is it possible,' I thought, 'that how I drive, is how I live?'. I clearly saw a correlation. Reflecting in the rear-view mirror of my life, I can honestly say, in all the times I 'tried' to force something or go against the flow, I crashed!

The perceived chaos on the roads here, really is an organised chaos. A chaos which isn't mine but what is mine is how I choose to handle it. React or respond? Driving and traveling through life is much easier and peaceful when responsive, allowing the natural ebb and flow. Flow brings order to chaos not just rules.

There will always be chaos on the roads and in life. I drive like a local now, creatively passing bikes and cars, both on the right and left, driving up onto sidewalks when traffic has come to a standstill and always getting myself safely from point A to point B. I acknowledge and accept when things are out of my control and practice mindfulness.

Living and driving from a place of confident assertion flows into enjoyment opposed to living and driving from a place of rigidity and reactivity.

There will always be detours and bumps on the roads and traveling through life. How we do one thing, is how we do everything, so loosen the rules from time to time, be flexible and open to experiencing something new, be creative, take a deep exhale, surrender to how things are 'supposed' to be and enjoy going with the flow.

YOU ARE NOT THE VOICES IN YOUR HEAD – YOU ARE NOT YOUR EXPERIENCES

Growing up, I always felt like a foreigner in my own country. A bit of a rebel really. I wasn't the labels society placed on me and I didn't desire the American Dream. I felt more at home traveling through foreign lands and being seen for who I was, rather than living a life I was 'supposed to' and told, would make me happy.

I was told I was different, as if that was a bad thing when really, I was just a girl with big dreams, who loved an adventure and wanted to explore the world.

As the years turned into decades, life events affected who I thought I was and I realised, I'd lost my way. It was looking into my own eyes, the windows of our soul and seeing a lifeless soul looking back, that my heart broke wide open. Pain often precedes peace and it was through my deepest pain that I met my true self.

With self-compassion and grace as my guides, I was able to surrender into stillness and learned to feel and express all the feelings that had been suppressed. I learned I wasn't my pain or the heaviness on my heart. I wasn't the voices in my head telling me I wasn't good enough, would always be angry and never escape the darkness of my shadows.

I wasn't the scars on my face, the cancer that had been in my body, nor the grief for all I'd lost or the dreams I'd left behind. I was not my feelings or my life experiences. Feelings came and went and my life experiences have strengthened my character.

I am not my age. I am divinely Me. My glorious self and sparkling at 60. I'm considered an elder and respected for the wisdom of my years. I'm a story teller standing in my truth, embracing the essence of who I am and who I am yet to become.

I am inspired and inspiring the women younger than I to continue to learn, create, grow and live their best lives. I am light. You are light. We are all light.

Celebrate YOU and the wisdom life has taught you.   Be gentle with yourself, embrace the essence of who you are and shine. Let the world see the sparkles in your eyes the messy hair and all that's in between.

BELIEVE IN YOURSELF - SEVEN LESSONS FROM AN IRONMAN (140.6 MILE SWIM, BIKE, RUN)

1. Know and respect your limits

If I was going to swim 2.4 miles, bike 112 miles and then run a marathon 26.2 miles, it had to be a scenic course with warm water, warm weather and relatively flat.

2. Character

Excitement may create momentum but a strong character is what gets us there.

3. Consistency

Show up and do your best even when you don't feel like it.

4. Ask and receive

It was so easy to ask for what I needed and receive it graciously. "What do you need?" asked the volunteers, always with a bright smile willing to support me in whatever I needed to run my race. From my favourites, the zipper strippers who were ready and waiting as I ran out of the water and into T1 (Transition 1) to unzip and pull me out of my wetsuit, to the woman who tied my runners to save me time, as I finished changing into my run kit, the boy who sprayed me down with sunblock, to the kind man who unwrapped and gave me a bite size chocolate I'd only been able to point to, my hands shaking as I slowed to walk through an aid station.

5. Smile and enjoy the compliments

I had just gotten out of the water, pulled my swim cap and goggles off when a spectator yelled out to me "Nice earrings!". I was touched, smiled into the crowd and thanked him. The next morning, my bestie surprised me with the paper. I'd made the front page. There I was, in black and white with my gold earrings, smiling into the crowd!

6. Celebrate

I was overwhelmed with emotion when I saw the red carpet. I wanted to savour every moment, knowing I would only cross the Finish Line of my first Ironman, once in a lifetime. When my foot hit the carpet I did the unexpected. I blew kisses to the crowd, throwing my arms in the air shouting "Yes, yes, yes!". The crowd went wild cheering me on and then I heard, Mike Reilly's infamous voice over the loud speaker, "Mikel Ann Hall from San Diego, CA – You are an Ironman!"

7. Never give up on your dreams

Always believe. You'll be amazed at what you accomplish!

WE DON'T REALISE HOW STRONG WE ARE UNTIL BEING STRONG IS OUR ONLY CHOICE

Growing up on the bright sunny beaches of southern California, sunblock was used as an after-thought, while baby oil was lavishly applied to my fair skin, in the hopes of sporting a golden tan.

I never did sport that golden tan. Instead I've visited a dermatologist's office every six months and recently every month. Skin damage was done and continues to emerge. Most visits are painful as pre-cancerous cells are frozen and burned off.

Skin cancer sucks. It's brought me to my knees on multiple occasions and placed me in the operating theatre under a knife, three different times in eighteen months. The pain I've endured stripped my character to the core. When I felt I couldn't go on and lost the will to live, I found hope and comfort in God's love. It's been a deep process of grief, of loss, of holding on tightly, trying to control, fix and escape the discomfort and has been exhausting. I was living in a state of 'I want to but I can't'. I literally didn't have the capacity and my nervous system froze, shut down and disconnected.

Only from a place of utter collapse, was I able to surrender. It's here that I learned how to meet my body where it was with gentleness, simplicity, less control, pressure or rush to change and to heal. I learned what no-one taught me, the nervous system heals in safety. Safety in the capacity to hold myself, mind-body energy in the midst of discomfort.

This journey has been a deeply painful one and one, I have come to accept and continue to walk. Choosing 'quiet' while my skin heals has taught me to choose me and respect where I'm at. It's deepened my self-compassion and grace. I'm now able to move through the trauma in a safe and empowering way.

Today, I am resilient, peaceful and deeply grateful for all that I've endured. It's been a gift in that it's taught me to show up for myself, to respect my body and that I'm a lot stronger than I think. Somehow I always find the courage to make the next appointment and the bravery to show up.

The only way out is through. Know that whatever you are going through you are stronger than you think.

PLACE YOUR HAND ON YOUR HEART, WHAT DO YOU FEEL?

A journey of unlearning and remembering. Letting go of stories and accepting the truth. It began with a request and a question. "Place your hand on your heart. What do you feel?" I felt nothing. What was I 'supposed' to feel? I hadn't a clue. I was disconnected from myself and from life.

Disconnection can be a response to trauma. We detach, freeze, deny and disappear into our minds, all in the name of survival. A strategy meant to be short term, had become my way of life. Through creating meaningful rituals, I was able to re-connect to myself, and discovered a deeper self-love and love for life again.

Mornings began in prayer and gratitude, honouring myself. Ceremonial cacao opened my heart. Breathwork softened it and gave me the courage to sit with the silence and feel the scary bits. I began exploring the shadows and parts I'd been unwilling and not able to sit with.

I got curious and discovered a large tightly spun web of untruths. The theme, "I'm different from everyone else and not worthy of being seen or heard and was abandoned by many."

I listened to everything that came up, discerning truth from untruths. In time, I learned to see myself for who I am and made myself a promise. I would accept and love all of me. After all, we are all different and uniquely and wonderfully made.

I learned the deepest pain came from within. By believing and living in untruths, I was the one not seeing or hearing myself. I was the one abandoning myself, not others.

Today when I place my hand on my heart, I feel. I feel love. I'm aware of my breath and feel blessed for the essence of who I am, a colourful mosaic of simplicity and complexity, light, shadows and all shades in between.

"Close your eyes and place your hand on your heart. What do you feel?" If you don't feel anything, know you're okay. Accept it with no shame, judgement or having to fix it. Underneath it, is all that's been missed in life, lost, repressed, suppressed and forgotten.

Feeling all the feels can be scary, yet is a portal to healing and the beginning to re-connection. Take a deep breath in, exhale slowly and feel what's there.

Karen has re-invented herself,
she's asked for help when she
needed it and when life called her
to dig in deep and find her voice
she did.

"This book is a gift" says Karen,
she's felt able to use her voice in
words on the written page in this
chapter, just for you, so her words
may inspire you to find your voice
too.

Her wish is for you to feel strong,
know that you are good enough
and that you can be exactly who
you want to be!

@karen_pullan_yoga

KAREN PULLAN

RE-INVENT YOURSELF AS MANY TIMES AS YOU NEED TO

After college, I worked in a corporate environment for thirty-five years. I climbed the ladder to a leadership role but I wasn't happy. 'Miserable' probably best described how I felt every day.

Redundancy threats hung over my head for five years until finally, in my early fifties, I was out. I was completely exhausted. I'd had to make lots of people redundant too. I hated this part of my job, so many people had moved house, purchased their first home, started a family and I had the grotesque task of making them redundant!

I hated myself. I was tired and angry and I became poorly. I took six months out to decide what my next steps were and to recover.

I quickly decided never to work for anyone else again. I also thought no-one would want to employ a middle-aged woman with (what I thought were) no skills, so why even bother!

I knew my life was going to be very different. I already had a holistic and alternative mindset, I was a Reiki and Access Bars Practitioner. I took a degree (I have 'BSc (Hons) Psyche' after my name which pleases me!) and at fifty-four, I trained as a psychotherapeutic counsellor.

I had a personal yoga practice too and when my yoga teacher moved away, I thought 'Hell why not!' and at fifty-five I trained to be a yoga teacher, a meditation teacher, a breathwork coach and added Ayurveda training there too.

I've taught like crazy, honing my skills, becoming a trauma informed yoga teacher as well and now in my sixtieth year, I'm writing a chapter for a book and creating women's circles!

It's never too late to make changes and become who you want to be. You just have to have the confidence to take the first step.

DON'T BE AFRAID TO BE VULNERABLE AND ASK FOR HELP

Can you ask for help? I couldn't. OMG, I had to be able to do everything myself and the quest to be perfect? It was fucking exhausting!

I'd never let anyone help, even if I hurt myself mentally or physically, even if it cost me more money; I'd be sure to bloody well do it myself!

I considered asking for help to be a weakness, being vulnerable was a weakness; although interestingly, I never saw others as being weak if they needed help. This only applied to me! I must have really disliked myself. I only came to understand this, when I trained as a therapist. I understood that to be 'perfect', was to please my mother! I couldn't show any sign of weakness to her and I craved her praise (which was elusive) so I continued.

I didn't have the tools back then but I do now. My relationship with mum now is great; I don't try to please her or seek her words of pride. I know she's proud of me, I know she loves me...in her way. Maybe not how I need but she is doing her best. I'm only sad it took me fifty years before I recognised that. I could have had a much better relationship with her sooner if I had known that.

Do I ask for help now? Hell yes! Age (and therapy) has taught me that it actually makes life a little easier. Can I be vulnerable now? Hell yes –it shows I'm not super woman. I'm doing the best I can.

How do I feel? Pretty good! All I can do is my best and if it isn't good enough, then so be it. I only have myself to please and to be who I am.

Always, always ask for help. It makes the journey more enjoyable.

CHANGE YOUR PERSPECTIVE AND THE COMPANY YOU KEEP

I often used to think the world was shit. I'd struggled to find my place and had lots of words in my head telling me it was 'horrid', 'cruel', 'evil' even. I remember being angry a lot of the time, all I could see was this horrid place that I had to try to navigate.

I was like this for years and yet I was fortunate enough to travel extensively for most of my life. I've seen some amazing places and met the most beautiful of people and still, I was angry with the world. It wasn't until my late forties, that I realised not everyone saw the world that way! The more people I connected with, the more I actually listened, the more I found different perspectives. I'd surrounded myself with like-minded people who thought the way I did, it seemed we all had a downer on the world!

I started to spend less time with the 'nay tellers' and more with the people who saw beauty and OMG, was this a revelation! I started to change my outlook and see that, on the whole, people are beautiful, the world is actually a beautiful place! I saw it much more clearly when I left my self-destructing bubble.

It was like standing on a mountain top on a clear day, looking out as far as you can see...there's mountains, snow, green fields and rolling hills. There are rivers and streams and oceans, sandy beaches and pebble beaches.

To view from a place of clarity showed me just how beautiful it can be! Step away and let go of the negativity and the people who keep you there. Change your outlook and see the world as the beautiful place it is!

ENJOY YOUR OLDER YEARS

As I become older, I'm noticing some things...general aches and pains are more obvious, I guess as I age, these could become my topics of conversation in my nursing home!

I noticed that when I got up, it was followed by a groan and a 'She's up!' with a little cheer and while my 10k runs are gone, I do think getting older is a frame of mind.

I like the word 'retirement', it fills me with joy, knowing I don't have to go to work! I recently received a letter stating I could take my pension! That floored me somewhat. I phoned my mum (in her glorious eighties) "When the fuck did that happen!" I asked, she just laughed, "Go with it, you can't stop it! Don't spend time chasing your youth, it'll only make you miserable!".

Now I'm over the shock, retirement feels full of opportunities. All the things I wanted to do when I worked full time are now open and available to me. I can finally be me and enjoy myself - hell I could be here for another thirty years!

It's a space filled with new beginnings. A new chapter where I get to do what the hell I want! By the time you reach sixty, no-one's particularly interested in what you do and, to be fair, I don't give a monkeys' chuff what anyone thinks either.

I'm fully embracing my weirdness; I dance in the rain, I make snow angels in pure white snow and I get into swimwear on the beach without a care for my wobbles, dimples and saggy skin. Getting older is freeing, a time to expand, a happy place, it's one to be enjoyed. Go your own way and be true to yourself. Don't be afraid of getting older. It is indeed a gift.

IT'S OK TO CRY

I've cried because I'm happy, I've cried because I'm sad, I've cried at weddings, funerals and christenings. I've cried at TV programmes, I've cried at the news, I've cried when I've seen good friends and family again and I've cried when they've left.

Crying heals the darkest of places. Sometimes I've cried and cried until my eyes have felt like they're bleeding. My lungs have burned so much it felt as though they were on fire. Crying doesn't fix the problem...my parents and grandparents would say, 'it's pointless!'. Well...it might not fix anything but it bloody well ISN'T pointless!

Even through all the physical pain I've found myself in, it bloody well felt good to release the anger, frustration, fear or sadness. Overwhelm and anxiety clear when we cry, actual raw crying helps let go of all our shit – it's cathartic!

A beautiful way of letting go. Just like when it rains and washes away the dust and grime. Tears bring a renewed calm, a release of tension and a clearer lens on the world.

Cry as often as you need to. You'll find release, peace and eventually a way through some of the darkest parts of your life. It's ok to cry!

SPEAK UP UNTIL YOU'RE HEARD

I recently read that an unhealed person carrying decades of emotional pain has a distinct energy that others can almost feel their rage bubbling under the surface, from their needs that have gone unmet and their abandonment that hasn't been processed.

When I read this, I cried. This is me, this is fucking me! Feeling unheard for most of my life, being told to stay quiet much of the time as a child, they told me my mouth would get me into trouble...then I was accused of being a shy and quiet child...it's no fucking wonder!

I too was raging on the inside, desperate to speak and to be heard. For fifty plus years, I was in this state, through childhood and later in an abusive marriage, where I was told I was worthless and that I had nothing of value to say. I was well and truly fucking raging! I bit my tongue at work, swallowing down my words. I controlled what was going on inside me, a ticking timebomb.

Fortunately, when I trained in psychotherapy, I went through lots of therapy myself and finally felt heard. 'Heard' and 'listened to' are different to me, 'heard' is deeper and has more connection. 'Listened to' doesn't have connection. Being heard, for me is more about being seen, being witnessed and having some validation that I was ok, that I was valuable, that I had a voice and I could be heard.

Don't ever be afraid to speak up, say what you want to say – always. It may fall on deaf ears but at some point someone will truly hear you. When you find these people, keep them close. If you need to, go to therapy to be heard – GO!

SELF-CARE ISN'T SELFISH

'I don't have time', 'I have to do...', 'I'm too busy'... I hold my hand up, I've said them and I have a long list of reasons why I can't take time for self-care.

'Self-care' isn't selfish though. It's about being and doing what makes you feel happy and good. It's important to your mental well-being, it's good for the soul!

Self-care is actually being able to say 'no!'...without justification! I used to think that doing all the things, then dropping myself in the bath at the end of the day was self-care! Maybe you do to? But why are we bottom of the list? Let go of 'shoulds', they're not yours. They're the things you believe you need to do, Which, if you think about it, came from someone else's list!

Whose voice are you hearing? Your mother, grandmother, aunt? 'Shoulds', instill themselves into our minds, picking away at us, putting us down! Start changing your sentences. You might start saying 'I should do the washing...' but finish saying 'but I'm not going to!'. Progress to 'I'm going to do (insert self-care plan)' instead.

You might even find yourself at 'I'm doing what I need right now for me, fuck that other shit!'. Do all the things you love more often! Let go of people or situations that drain you. Say no without justification. Doodle. Close your eyes. Breathe in. Listen to songs. It's your life. Do what you need.

VALUE YOURSELF, SET BOUNDARIES, KEEP REAL FRIENDS CLOSE

I believe that valuing yourself, means having boundaries. And if you create boundaries, not everyone will like it...in fact...most won't and they're likely to tell you, you've changed. Authentic friends, real friends, the ones your heart trusts and the ones whose intentions are genuine, will like you for who you are regardless of your need to set boundaries.

I had a time when I was so scared to lose friends and acquaintances, people who didn't always have the best of intentions for me. I actually didn't really like myself much; how could I expect anyone else to like me? My boundaries changed which was confusing and it was exhausting. I wore so many masks. I started to create small boundaries, like being able to say 'no'. 'No!' is actually a full sentence and needs no further justification.

Each time I introduced a new boundary, the next would become easier. I found people melting away, my circle became smaller but I was more comfortable and happier. I had people who wanted to be with me.

Choose your life partner well. Make sure you'd like them as a friend. Would they hold your hair back when you puke? Choose someone who'll clean up the mess with you when life gets hard, someone who'll support your life choices, even if they don't agree.

Surround yourself with people who put effort in to be around you. Don't be the one to chase. Supporters and encouragers want to be around us, they inspire us to be better versions of ourselves. Take time to find these people, they're looking for you too.

As a once-shy child, Janine continually surprises herself by finding the courage within to speak her truth and challenge authority when necessary. She raises her voice often for those who cannot.

Her two daughters constantly inspire her to discover and speak her truth.

Guided by her intuition, Janine challenged herself to put her wisdom into words and express her deepest thoughts, in the hope that you, dear reader, find your own wisdom.

"Be reassured" she says, "we all have our own journey and life struggles but it's not what happens to us, it's how we choose to deal with the situation that really matters".

@makesperfectscents_holistic

JANINE VINE

LET GO OF RELATIONSHIPS THAT WEIGH YOU DOWN

I'd love to say that I breezed through my early fifties, sadly, I didn't. I was supposed to feel fifty and fabulous, so why didn't I? I was at a crossroads, feeling stagnant, no energy or enthusiasm. I had ground to a halt.

It was time to change lanes from the road to nowhere, back onto the highway of happiness. My GPS recalibrated, I set the destination to positivity. So changing gears, I waved goodbye to people and relationships that weighed me down, almost as if they were the flat tyres of my old wheels lying by the side of the road. As I freed myself from these connections, I felt a sense of space within me opening, allowing my creativity and passion to blossom once more. Slowly but surely, jealousy and small mindedness faded into my rear-view mirror, while those who inspired me illuminated my path. There's a saying, 'Tell me who your friends are and I'll tell you who you are!'.

My new direction was towards a tribe that matched my vibe. A beautiful close-knit circle of like-minded kindred spirits who uplifted, encouraged and supported me and I them.

Together we embarked on a heartfelt quest to become our truest, authentic selves. I've learned over the years, not to be impressed by material wealth but rather to be enriched in life by kindness, wisdom and deep connections. This transformative journey is only the start.

In finding my tribe, I found my true path and reset my course and there is so much more to come.

Darling if you find yourself here at the crossroads, scared but brave, I ask you to stop and listen to your heart. Trust in this new journey, it may just take you on the ride of your life.

CELEBRATE YOUR AGE, FORGET THE STEREOTYPES

As a child, I often dreamed of having super powers and being invisible. Oh the irony! Be careful what you wish for!

I'd happily trade a Harry Potter Invisibility cloak for a snazzy pair of bifocals. I've been witness to ageism, it's a thing, especially for women and it's high time we did something about it.

If we could just remove prejudice and discrimination; disrupt the stereotype that women are no longer useful or relevant over a certain age. I've learned that ageing isn't about fading into the background, it's about growing and blossoming into the best version of ourselves. We're just like trees in nature. We stand proud and firmly rooted, we weather storms, adapt to change and instead of leaves, we sprout wisdom and life lessons.

Ageing is indeed a privilege that sadly not everyone gets to experience, embrace it with open arms my love. We all age, regardless of gender or race. It's not exclusive and how we handle it, is entirely in our hands.

Celebrate your age, your positive ageing experience with those younger and revel in your wisdom!

APPRECIATE THE INNER CHILD IN YOU

Dear Inner Child,

I've been thinking about you lately and wanted to take a moment to tell you how much I cherish that magical playful spirit you embody.

I know for a short while, we lost touch with each other. It wasn't your fault dearest one, it was mine. I was too busy focusing on the stresses of life, I was no longer living, merely existing.

As I reflect, I realise how I missed your wide-eyed curiosity, how you'd seek out the wonders in every single day, exploring new ways to do what you love, turning ordinary moments into extraordinary adventures.

Rediscovering the art of playfulness has reminded me of the joys of being silly. I goof around now unapologetically and I laugh so hard, tears run down my face, surely, there's no better tonic to soothe one's soul?

We must embrace this playground of life together. As George Bernard Shaw once said, 'We don't stop playing because we grow old, we grow old because we stop playing'.

Over the years, I've learned to combine the wisdom I've gained with your boundless imagination, creating a synergy that continues to guide me. I promise to honour your spirit and nurture your presence within me.

Your light shines so brightly, it radiates through me like a glorious sunbeam. Without you, I can't reach for the stars. You, my dear, hold the key to a more vibrant and authentic life and when I'm with you, I'm home.

LOVE YOUR NAKED BODY

As I stand naked, gazing at my reflection in the mirror, I'm reminded of the youthful figure that once was. This wasn't sadness I felt but regret.

It's funny how I'm so quick to correct my daughters, when they talk negatively about their bodies, yet I failed to take my own advice when I was younger. Journeying through my fifties, I learned valuable lessons about the relationship I have with my body. This beautiful vessel has grown and nurtured two children and allowed me to experience the joys of life. It's kept me going, even through the toughest of times.

The lines on my face reflect all the smiles and laughter, the dimpling on my thighs is the result of many a delicious cake and conversation with good company. Why would I deny myself that?

Our bodies show evidence that we have lived! They've carried us through life with grace and strength. So, I've ditched the narrative that looking a certain way will make me happier, more loved or help me gain approval from my peers, because it doesn't.

Our bodies are not a valid measure of our value as individuals. We all come in different shapes and sizes and body confidence, most definitely, comes from within. Embrace your beautiful uniqueness darling, speak kindly to yourself and make peace. Your body deserves your gratitude, don't make it wait for your love.

MENOPAUSE PASSES

My mother may well have seen the signs had she still been alive, God love her but sadly, she had passed. When I think back to when she was a similar age, I don't recall any such thing. That said, I was far too busy being a teenager.

My mother was brought up in a Convent where I'm sure the order of the day was to suffer in silence. I myself had never previously suffered with as much as a headache before my mid-forties, so when bombarded with brain fog, insomnia and debilitating migraines, the doctors failed to see the signs and there was cause for concern. Unbeknownst to me, I'd entered new uncharted territory of the delightful 'perimenopause'. I thought I was quite literally losing my marbles; it was terrifying.

Finally at fifty-eight and after thirteen years in a rollercoaster of emotions, I am done! I've taken Menopause quite literally on the chin, good news beards are in! Who knew this was something hubby and I would experience together in the mornings. Razor anyone?

Joking aside, menopause is a natural life transition, not to be feared, just better understood!

NEVER TOO LATE: THE SECOND ACT 'THE GOLDEN AGE OF POSSIBILITIES'

For many years, my family were the centre of my entire universe. Watching my daughters grow into amazing women, filled me with pride. Now they've flown the nest and my focus has shifted towards pursuing my own dreams.

Looking back, I realise I'd prioritised the needs of others, placing my own goals and passions on hold. At the time I was quite content cheering on from the side-lines while others shone. I don't regret my decisions, the road less travelled has led me here to this moment, writing this chapter.

Taking that all-important leap of faith though and starting something new, takes courage. I've had complete faith in my intuition, so I've just jumped right in, trusting the net would appear. It's quite exhilarating and somewhat empowering that I've finally turned the page, I'm excited to see where this next chapter takes me!

Call me a 'late bloomer' but I've always loved the appearance of an unexpected rose in Autumn and as I sit here writing, I'm reminded of a quote by CS.Lewis, 'You're never too old to set another goal or to dream a new dream'.

The power in such simple yet poignant words, they've become my daily mantra. Don't allow the voices inside your head to tell you it's too late. Own your awesomeness and show the world your beautiful uniqueness...greatness has no expiration date!

DITCH THE OVER THINKING, YOU DON'T NEED IT

I have to confess, I'm the 'Queen of Overthinking'. In fact, if it were an Olympic sport, I'd definitely have gained a gold medal or two. But here's the thing. All that overthinking left me feeling behind and full of missed opportunities. I slowly came to realise that procrastination, for me, was just another word for fear and actually, that stemmed from deeper issues.

I'd overthink every single detail, happily putting things off or even worse, not attempting them at all. You see where I'm going with this? Yes, absolutely nowhere! I'm not going to lie, it's hard to break habits you've had for an entire lifetime but sure enough, those small steps forward were better than none.

I realised the only way to achieve my goals was to take action and break the cycle. It was time the Queen of Overthinking dethroned herself and took back control of her life. I've learnt that 'done' is better than 'perfect', as it's those little imperfections that make life more interesting and worth living. And if all else fails, remember, there's always tomorrow or the next day or the day after that! (just kidding!)

ALWAYS QUESTION HOW YOU LABEL YOURSELF

I used to be a self-proclaimed 'technophobe'. I clung to my Motorola like it was a precious artefact, refusing to upgrade to an iPhone out of fear that I wouldn't be able to keep up with the latest technology. It felt like everyone was speaking a different language and I was lost in translation.

Thanks to my daughters and their persistence, I finally took the plunge and joined the digital age. Although, I must confess, my new iPad remained unopened for a couple of months before I plucked up the courage to start.

The thought of having to learn what others had had a lifetime to perfect, in such a short space of time, just to keep up, was somewhat overwhelming. Slowly but surely, I persevered, embracing a growth mindset and switching my identity from 'technophobe' to 'tech enthusiast'. I had labelled myself and I re-labelled myself too.

I've learned that questioning my identity and my limiting beliefs, has allowed me to discover new passions and life skills. I'm glad to say I'm no longer stuck in the dark ages and while I'm by no means a tech-wizard, I am optimistic about the future and living proof that you can teach an old dog a few new tricks!

Numerous women have inspired Jenn to find her voice. "Too many to mention" she says. However, she believes her cancer diagnosis really pushed her to live life on her own terms.

She learned that playing small and compromising didn't make her happy. Instead, understanding herself, connecting to her inner wisdom and courage, gave her the permission she needed to speak up. Sharing her thoughts initially with a small tribe of like-minded women, empowered her to express herself in all areas.

She was compelled to write her chapter so others could learn from her experiences. "I would have loved a book like this! Encountering such powerful, insightful words of wisdom from women could have made such a difference for me... in so many ways".

@radiant.real.women.jenn.levers

JENN LEVERS

LIVE WILD!

I was a wild child, a rebel, a 'bad girl'. Inquisitive, with boundless energy, I was probably a nightmare for my parents, forever in trouble, my exuberant energy would take over and before I knew it, I was in a dilemma!

Adults and authority figures told me to be quiet, sit still, 'stop it!'. I remember being told 'I should be ashamed of myself' and that I didn't know how to behave. I thought that meant there was something wrong with me.

I spent adulthood hiding the real me for fear of humiliation and embarrassment yet now I realise – it was an exuberance of life that I had...something to celebrate!

It was the wild woman in me, my love and joy, wanting to be 'out there' in the world. That wildness? It was me...it was all me!

It took getting into my fifties with some life-changing experiences under my belt to realise I missed that wildness I'd tamed, my exuberance and love for life. That side of me was desperate to be out there again! So now...I'm embracing all of me, I'm celebrating ME!

My whimsical nature, my joy for my friends and quirky sense of humour, my need to travel and explore. My love of nature, my own company, food, sea and forests! I desire to make a difference, I have courage and compassion!

Awaken the wild side in you, your wild woman. Listen to the adventures that call, celebrate you! Dance, live wild and free. Emerge from your chrysalis – it's time to fly. Release the freedom from within, melt into the love of life and own that wild side of you...LIVE! LIVE! LIVE!

ONLY YOU CAN TRULY LOVE AND PLEASE YOURSELF

Until a few years ago, I wasn't sure who I was. I felt as if I'd been living someone else's life rather than mine.

I'd worn so many masks to fit in, I'd become so good at pleasing that I could walk into any situation and fit in. I was able to be whatever I needed to be in any given situation. This was so all-consuming, I lost sight of 'me'.

I didn't know what was important to me, how to love myself or accept myself, I didn't know who I was! When my father died...it all changed. It hit me hard with a deep wrenching away of all that had been familiar to me. I'd been living my life for dad's validation, playing a role to make him proud, looking for him to validate me and show me love.

Life became so much easier when I let that go and just became myself. I realise now that finding this 'deep knowing' of me was so profound, I learned the difference between pleasing myself and pleasing another. It's where my wisdom lives, it's where my freedom lives, it's where your freedom lives too.

Look in the mirror every day. Say to yourself 'I love you!'. It may feel strange but just wait until the day you can believe it fully and receive it fully. That's true freedom!

STOP COMPARING YOURSELF TO OTHERS

Comparing yourself to others never achieves what you want it to. I used to do this until I realised one day, it was doing me no good! I was either comparing from a place of judging the other person for how they looked (to give me a boost) or I was coming from a place of poor comparison...of not feeling good enough and not measuring up!

Neither is a great way of being. We're all unique and beautiful in our own way. We undermine our own power every time we ignore ourselves and look to others for how we should look, how we should feel and how we should behave. We ignore our own truths, our wants and our desires. We undermine our own power when we compare from a place of fear. Fear that we are somehow lacking, unworthy or undeserving.

We undermine our power every time we compare ourselves to others, not trusting who we are and not respecting ourselves and we undermine ourselves with comparisons that ignore how awesome and amazing we really are!

Remember you are unique.
No one else can do what you can do.
No one else can be what you are!

The sun and the moon are completely different entities but they both shine brightly. Shine as you. Be you. Be your RADIANT REAL Self.

IT IS YOUR RESPONSIBILITY TO MAKE YOU HAPPY, NO-ONE ELSE'S

It's not anyone else's responsibility to make you happy. It's a waste of time to put the responsibility of your happiness anywhere else but with you. Different people and circumstances can bring you joy, yes but they aren't where your true happiness comes from. You can waste a great deal of energy looking to things in your life to make you happy.

True happiness doesn't come from your job, your family, your friends or partner, it comes from inside, the way you view the world. You and you alone, are in charge of building your own happiness.

I've worked at it. I've changed jobs, countries, and partners. I've moved house so many times, my mum bought a new address book just for me! I've flitted between friendships and none of those outside elements created any real, deep lasting happiness. It's how I was inside that mattered. My perspective on what was happening around me.

Forgive yourself, stop replaying what should have been, find ways to accept. Let go of grievances that happened years ago, they will only sour your life today.

Believe in your power to make yourself happy, you are so much more able to do this than you think. Make inner peace and your own happiness a priority.

Smile at yourself in the mirror, laugh for no reason and spend time towards the end of each day self-reflecting and meditating. Melt into loving, relaxing and slowing down in the knowledge that everything is going to be ok. You can be happy.

YOU ARE NOT RESPONSIBLE FOR HOW THOSE AROUND YOU FEEL

Please don't compromise who you are for someone else. In my early thirties, I was with a man who was probably very insecure. I frequently felt undermined. He had this beautiful, intelligent, quirky woman on his arm, he liked to be seen with her but he couldn't control her.

I'm almost ashamed to admit it, I thought it was my fault. I let him chip away at my self-esteem and confidence. On my birthday one year, I wanted to look sexy; I bought a little black dress. I knew I looked good in it, so I walked into the lounge, stood in front of him and waited for him to tell me I looked beautiful. He looked me up and down, made a non-committal noise and told me I looked ridiculous. He said he didn't want to be seen in public with me!

I started wearing baggy clothes, covering up, dressing down, hiding my body and my sexiness...after all, I didn't want to upset him!

It was only when a good friend said he was worried about me, that he'd lost the person he knew and that I didn't smile anymore, that I realised I'd taken responsibility for how my partner felt. I had to realise it was ok for me to wear a beautiful dress and feel beautiful.

Of course, I left the relationship. I cleared out my wardrobe...everything was baggy tops and jumpers, clothes I'd hidden in. It was such a great feeling to throw them out. I started a new wardrobe...one that reflected me! One that allowed me to shine.

Always keep sight of who you are and never base your self-worth on someone else. Walk away if you need to but always shine your light!

WRITE YOUR OWN RULES

Looking back over the years, I see I tried to live my life following other people's rules...rules I thought I had no choice but to follow.

I lived life with a deep fear that I may not be up to the mark, that I might fail or not be accepted. I kept the persona of 'fun-loving Jenn' with a smile on her face, the good girl, the perfect friend, the perfect partner, the perfect daughter all without realising I didn't have to do that. You know, nothing happens if you remove those masks!

Over the years, I wrote my own rules for life, it's so empowering! I set the way for others too, showed them it was ok not to follow the rules. Decide what your own rules are, what your values are and live by those.

I have to show up as me now...always! So please, just show up as you. Write your own rules about how you want to behave. Throw away the masks you've hidden behind, the convenient rules...throw them all away.

Live by your own expectations of you! Conform to your idea of you!

IT'S NEVER TOO LATE TO LIVE THE LIFE YOU WANT

I started my life story well actually...travelling...really experiencing the world. A real sense of freedom, a real sense of me, who I was and what I wanted to be.

I got a little lost in the middle, I allowed my desire for adventure to slip away somehow. Nothing major happened, I just allowed other things to become more important. My job took over, earning money, buying a house, buying a car...the desire for possessions...they all took over...and adventure was forgotten.

My cancer diagnosis and the threat of losing my life made me realise my story wasn't finished! I'd been surviving life but not thriving!

It was time to start living again! I had so many more chapters to write, so many more adventures to experience. Imagine you're an author, the author of your story. The author of your life.

Who would be in your life? What would you do with your day? Where would you put your energy? What adventures would you have? What would the next chapter look like? What would happen next?

Move towards what motivates you, what fills you with energy. Be grateful for all that you have every day. Do what makes you feel most alive! Travel, gain life experience, love unconditionally and follow what sets you on fire and flames your spirit!

Keep moving, keep dancing, playing and laughing. Be the author of your life. Live like this is the best time of your life, no matter what you do. Re-write your life from where you are now. Exciting eh!

IT'S NOT ABOUT HOW YOU LOOK, IT'S ABOUT THE ENERGY YOU RADIATE

My twenties were all about my looks, how sexy I was, how clear my skin was. My hair had to look good...Oh, the amount of hairspray I used!

My breasts were beautiful, my legs were shapely and I had to be slim! I put so much effort and money into my looks, most of my friends did too, we were all very fashion conscious. I used to look at all the major fashions and buy material for a pound a yard at Birmingham's Rag market in my lunchtime and copy their creations...lots of punk style clothes based on Vivienne Westwood's wonderful styles.

Much has changed in my life since those times. Having had a radical mastectomy, I've had to come to terms with many things...my new body shape...the reflection in the mirror...the scars...

The biggest adjustment? The realisation that people don't actually respond to how you look...they respond to the energy you radiate, what shines through from inside!

It took me over a year to realise that one! For much of that year, I couldn't look at myself, I hated what I saw - the disfigurement, the ugliness, the loss of my identity as a woman. I hid away in total shame. I also realised, however, that I'd hidden away even before my operation, so I hadn't been happy then either!

Gradually, acceptance and love for myself, replaced uncertainty and loss. I began to see an inner radiance in me, an inner beauty. For the first time, it wasn't about how I looked.

Despite losing a breast, I am the happiest I've been for a long time about my body. Not because I'm prettier or thinner but because I totally accept me and my inner beauty. My energy makes me shine, not my body!

People will always be drawn to your light, your energy, your inner radiance...how you carry yourself and how it feels to be around you. People will accept and love you for exactly who you are.

Step into your power! This is your age of possibility! The age of the RADIANT REAL you.

A mother and a grandmother, she
is finally writing her words. A
legacy for the future, she is seeing
herself as the writer and author
she is, finding the voice that wasn't
always heard in the past.

Surrounded by a supportive and
inspirational circle of friends, she
is nurturing herself, reclaiming her
power and finding the next version
of her Self.

Writing this chapter has been a
clearing and a healing - she hopes
you find that in yourself too.

@thejoyfuljotter

JOY WEBB

ONLY KEEP A FRIENDS SECRET IF IT FEELS GOOD

They say you're a true friend if you keep and carry another's secret. Now, we all know loyalty, trust and shared secrets are part of real and deep friendship. But what if the weight of carrying someone else's darkest secret takes over your life? What if the keeping safe of another's secret extinguishes your light?

For many years, I carried the secret of a good friend. I watched as they bowed under the weight of what they considered a shameful secret. I looked on as they felt it and lived with it.

In my acceptance of their situation and my compliance to keep their secret, I felt like I lost my own identity. I would lie for them, cover up for them, hide it for them. But, try as I might, the person involved would not, could not, be helped.

In thinking, believing even, that I was protecting them, I absorbed their secret.

Like the imposter baby cuckoo in another bird's nest, their secret began to steal my dreams bit by bit as I adapted to holding it, making more and more space for it.

The day came when I felt I could no longer carry it. There was no more space for their secret. I had to allow my friend to take some shared responsibility for their secret as my spark for life dimmed.

I suppose it was a deep knowledge of what I needed to do to survive, for my own self-protection.

In the lifting of this heavy weight I'd be carrying and in the relief of being able to shine myself, I made space and light for my own dreams to come true and they broke free! The result is, I achieved my dream to write a book.

So, my love, if you're carrying someone else's secret, stop and ask yourself why. How much does it take from you and how heavy does it feel? You're allowed to let it go and lighten up your own life once more.

Don't ever be afraid to cry

"Don't cry", they said. "You're too sensitive" they said. "You take things way too personally". I'd heard these criticisms so many times as a child, I believed them. As a grown-up, being emotional, feeling emotional or showing emotion was deemed by those around me as 'my overreaction'. I've always been told not to feel things so deeply.

And so, for far too many years, I didn't cry my tears of wonder at the sunrise, the sunset, the first spring flowers, the glorious rainbows or the breath-taking ever-changing landscape of the sea.

I couldn't cry at the beautifully mellow autumn or the snow-covered trees. My uncried, untried tears fermented within me. They caused blockages mentally, I had 'brain fog' and attachment issues. Emotionally (through unexpressed grief and anger), I found myself physically ill and spiritually unwell by looking outside of my soul for peace.

Now I'm older, I cry. A lot! Crying and feeling into sensitivity is my absolute fuckin' SUPERPOWER! Now, by allowing sensitivity into my life, not being ashamed of tears and feeling everything, I've gained the confidence to be my real self. Sensitivity, I have discovered, is a friend who brings her sisters along for the ride too: empathy, intuition and kindness. They all gather round Sensitivity and assist her.

Don't ever be ashamed or frightened to cry, it means that you feel deeply. I do. Sensitivity and her sisters hold me close, I am safe with them. You will be too.

Get the tattoos or piercings if you want to, it's your body!

Over twenty years ago, I played it safe and had a discreet Chinese symbol tattooed on my right shoulder. I worked in the corporate world then, such things were frowned upon. And despite some people who said it might well have said 'curry and egg fried rice' I loved it! And I wanted another one.

I was talked out of it though by the frowns and unspoken displeasures of others. I heard comments like,

"Only sailors have tattoos"
"Only ears should be pierced"
"What will you look like when you're sixty? Ridiculous, that's what!"

Others expressed their disapproval and I listened until the urge to rebel took over me. I didn't want to be the 'good girl' anymore, I wanted to claim my body back!

As I approach sixty, I've fulfilled my wish and have three prominent tattoos I'm proud of. I've reclaimed my body for me and that feels good! Who knows what my next one will be! Stamp your feet, have a tantrum if you must but don't wait, say 'fuck you' and do it anyway!

DRESS FROM YOUR FEET UP

I have a saying 'A woman should always dress from her feet up!'. Your feet are what you use every day, they keep you rooted, connected to Mother Earth, grounded.

Years ago, in the corporate world, the dress code for women was a suit and heels! Uncomfortable, pinched toes that rubbed, sore heels and blisters...all for the sake of making Jimmy Choo's bank balance larger and looking lady-like in my profession!

Later on, I worked in factories, portacabins and freezing cold offices where warm socks and boots were far more practical, wellies were my favourite choice of footwear!

So, dress from your feet up. Trust me, your day will flow more easily and comfortably. My footwear of choice now are flip flops and sandals or even better, nothing at all. There's so much to be said for barefoot walking.

And don't get me started on my next piece of advice...big knickers! They're the icing on the cake in the comfort department, the second floor of dressing upwards from your feet!

And if you can't or 'don't do' big knickers and you're uncomfortable...well, you can always take them off...no one will know!

YOUR POWER IS IN YOUR PAUSE

I was designed and programmed to stop and rest. My ancestors knew that. They followed the seasons of nature and the cycles of the sun, moon, and stars.

As I got older, despite what the world told me, I knew I couldn't keep going, pushing on through, 'win the day' every day. I felt it in my bones and muscles, my digestion, I needed to pause and slow down. Stop rushing here, there and everywhere. It's ok to stop, pause and take a rest.

I really wish someone had told me that earlier, as life got busier. Extremely long working hours and high expectations, I expected to thrive on less sleep than I needed. A twenty-four-hour culture became my norm, eroding precious sleep. An overworker, I pushed myself to the limit. I was so tired but I couldn't admit it.

Even if you feel that deep and real change isn't possible for you at this very moment, don't give up on your dream of a life of flow and ease.

Take small steps towards a pause – allow yourself time every day for a walk, to write in a journal, to read a few pages of a book or take a bath.

Practice yoga, meditate if you can. Ten minutes if nothing else. Allow yourself some space to pause and breathe – deeply. You never know what change might come out of this.

YOUR BODY IS BLOODY AMAZING!

Over the years, the insecurity of not seeing myself as photogenic or attractive enough to keep up with the latest fashions meant that the true me was hidden. I hid myself beneath layers of cosmetics, unnecessary stuff that big corporates insisted I needed. Apparently, 'I was worth it'...or rather 'my money' was worth their advertising fees.

Please know that your body is absolutely bloody amazing! How others think you should look is NOT who you truly are inside, it's not who your essence or soul is. Buying into the consumerism (and advertising) of mass-produced chemical products to solve your 'perceived' flaws masks your actual true self. You and your body are good enough as they are.

Your true Self with your unique wrinkles, saggy bits and skin type...your body shape, your not-so-perfect teeth and hair are the vessel in which your real Self lives. I don't own a TV now. I don't read newspapers or magazines and I scroll past fashion and anti-ageing advertising. And you know why? Because putting on my favourite jeans and dressing for my Self is an act of rebellion. No make up one day, full face the next and nature provides in so many ways – there's nothing some coconut oil can't sort out!

Be kind to your body, mind and soul. Please don't compare yourself to the impossibly airbrushed fake images that bombard you from every angle. Their sole purpose is to make you feel insecure, spend your hard-earned cash and crush your soul.

True beauty comes from deep within your Soul. It's reflected in your smile, your kindness, your humility, your integrity. See yourself as others see you – as the beautiful, radiant vessel you are.

TIME IS A HUMAN INVENTION

We divide our days up into hours, minutes and seconds. On January 1st, we look at our newly gifted calendar for the next twelve months and think we have a whole year to do things, to become a 'new' version of ourselves. By 1st February, resolutions have fizzled out. Anniversaries and birthdays are celebrated as each year passes and yet, time does not actually exist in such a rigid format. The clock and calendar are human inventions that literally control and dictate our every waking hour.

In nature, 'time' passes in cycles and they don't have exact or precise boundaries. The seasons come and go...a week or two early...or late, the universe moves in sweeping grand cycles, as the sun, moon and earth dance around each other...in heavenly right timing.

The sun and moon choreograph this dance, moving and directing ocean tides and women's bodies...universal timing is powerful! Listen to and observe the general ebb and flow of life. Don't force things, you're not running out of time and it's never, ever too late.

Start something, end something, change something. We rush through life chasing deadlines and commercial seasons but all things happen in divine timing, not human timing.

Slow down, see the precious moments of joy, insight, quiet, learning and inspiration, they're all there, ebbing and flowing in divine timing!

Don't spend your life carrying guilt

When I was nearly five years old, my mother died. Suddenly. Abruptly. One morning she was there and by the end of the same day, she wasn't. I never saw her again. And I can't remember anyone ever telling me she wasn't coming back.

I knew from an early age that I was, in some fundamental way, different. I was different at school, in my workplaces, in my friendship circles... everywhere in life, really. Being a motherless daughter has been a lonely place. A deep loneliness within my heart that radiates to my physical body some days. Even now.

But the guilt I felt as a child has always been difficult for others to understand. No-one told me it was my fault but no-one told me it wasn't either. I believed I must have done something terribly wrong and I couldn't tell anyone.

Now, over fifty years later, with the help and support of friends and healing sessions, I understand that 'being different' is my story. I can't change it.

In accepting the shame and guilt, I'm now released from it and this gives me the confidence to tell my stories of childhood loss.

Carrying guilt of any kind slowly eats away at you from inside and affects your life and your well-being. It can make you feel unworthy, lack confidence in your true Self and your abilities. It weighs heavier and heavier in your heart as the years go by.

One day, you won't be able to carry it any longer and you'll gently put that burden down. Please don't spend your life carrying guilt. Set yourself free. Share it and release it.

Prem's inner child has been a source
of inspiration, urging her to use her
voice as a woman.

It's this voice that has propelled her
beyond her comfort zones and
moved her career forward.

She's used her voice in so many
roles: as a wife, partner, mentor and
yoga teacher, not to mention as a
mother to three.

She encourages other women to
express themselves too through both
holding and gathering
in women's circles.

Writing this chapter presented an
opportunity to grow in a new
direction, to serve others by
collaborating with like-minded
women in a space where she could
be seen, heard and genuinely
understood.

@premdevil08_in_cornwall

PREM DEVI

SHOULD I STAY OR SHOULD I GO?

Leaving someone I loved was one of the hardest things I've done. I'd stay up night after night mulling it over, 'should I stay or should I go?'.

I had no idea of love language or attachment styles, I just knew I loved him but I'd lost myself in that relationship, living his life, I became very anxious, I didn't know myself anymore.

I knew him very well, he was charming, made me laugh, was full of life and inspiration but my anxiety was rising and my self-esteem lowering. I had to be so brave, I put on my big girl pants and made the decision to end the relationship.

Some kind of relief came over me in doing that. Then thousands of tears spilt, heartbreak followed, then mixed emotions...compassion, gratitude and eventually healing.

It seems our relationships can be our biggest teachers. I've learnt a lot about myself, feeling into my own light and shadow's, knowing my worth and my boundaries but most of all I learned that if you happen to you lose yourself in love, you can always come back home to yourself.

Loving yourself is...a safe and sacred space, where you can accept ALL of you unconditionally. A most precious gift that can abide in your heart and eventually allow for a more aligned love.

FORGIVE

I meditate. I sit quietly and find my answers there. Deep in meditation, I remembered a childhood wound. It seemed to come from nowhere and rocked my world. Unspoken words of resentment and hurt came into my mind. As a young teenager, my mum unknowingly and unwillingly caused me pain.

In my teens, I couldn't comprehend her actions but now, in my later years, I know she had her reasons. As this wound arose to be seen, my heart filled with remorse, deepened into compassion.

After that, came understanding and pride for the mother she was. I didn't see her strength when she was here. I wish I could have thanked her and shown her more love and appreciation in her living years. I believe though that healing continues even after life itself and it resides in our hearts. It's never too late to forgive.

I also reflected how my own actions as a mum took a similar route when my children were teenagers. I too, lived with the pain that my decision shook and changed their worlds.

We all have reasons why we do what we do. We don't intend hurting anyone, least of all the ones we love but sadly we often do. Sometimes it seems we have no choice, when we're hurting on the inside and longing for our own happiness.

I forgave my mum and, in time I forgave myself for my own choices. And so, the healing continues. It's ok to forgive.

ALL DREAMS CAN AND DO COME TRUE

I had it all and gave it all up. The family life and home, the security, the business. A heart wrenching decision. As I arrived at my friends and explained, she said "Have you lost your mind?". "Maybe", I replied "... but I've gained hope".

Being separated from my children was the hardest part. Bonds and hearts broken. Two years of emotional turmoil engulfed me, the separation and divorce impacted us all. Breast cancer struck and sent my life into turmoil too.

I didn't blame anyone except myself, the deep guilt that I had allowed to eat away at me. In that darkness, I found hope and I strongly believed I'd get through it.

Time and healing were needed for us all. I overcame my illness and in time, relationships and hearts began to heal. Hope showed me what can be overcome, what's important. My unconditional love for my children and the understanding that our minds are powerful tools helped me listen to my heart.

Trust yourself to make difficult choices. Have hope for a better future, you'll be amazed how the universe supports you.

As my journey continues, I embrace hope and support, a divine flow keeps me growing into my fullest potential and living my best life. Now I fully trust in my intuition and in my heart. Recently, my intuition pulled me to make the three-hundred-mile road trip to surprise my daughter for her wedding dress fitting. Her reception of me was priceless; the love in that moment between us has been indented on my heart.

Darling, embrace all that arises in your heart, go for it and never give up hope that, in time, all dreams can and do come true.

BEING ALONE AND HAPPY

Most of us want to love and be loved. It can feel immensely beautiful and provide security but, as we spend much time searching for the one, we often by-pass the one inside us.

Two broken marriages and some unfulfilling relationships led me to delve into myself to find the one. Bruised and battered emotionally, it was time to dig deep and take a long hard look at myself. I actually felt like my inner child was smiling in delight that I'd chosen to come home.

Yoga and meditation helped me find my inner home. I found stillness and silence there and when I found that space, I found all the things...childhood pain, a few wounds, a way of releasing, a lot of courage and most importantly choice.

A Leo with a big heart, I'm known for my outgoing personality, passion and zest for life but inside, a soft, sensitive part of me needed to be felt, seen and heard.

How to feel into that place, while protecting myself, seemed impossible and yet, I finally have my own special inside space held in a valley to simply breathe deeply, relax or release. Sometimes I chant quietly or sing loudly, sometimes I dance wildly in my underwear, cook delicious food or simply just love being ME.

Being in love is wonderful but being in love with myself is God damn empowering!

FEAR CANNOT SURVIVE WHERE COURAGE RESIDES

Fear is my shadow friend; it appears often gripping my chest, catching my breath. I see it as testing my courage, my strength and my growth. Many times, I've given in to fear and let someone help me out. There's no shame in that, sometimes it's even the stepping stone I need to then go on and do things alone.

When it arrives these days, I recognise it and embrace it. I breathe deeply with my hand on my heart, allowing each slow breath to soothe my nervous system. I find that process allows space for my courage to rise and move into the space where my fear was.

I also have a belief that I'm never alone. Even though I'm alone physically, I don't believe I'm alone spiritually. When I feel fear, I ask the divine angels to be beside me and protect me.

Visiting new places and walking alone has held fear for me but often, when I bring courage in and ask my angels for protection, I get the joy of meeting interesting new people and, as it happens, they're often alone too. The real gem I find, is the freedom and liberation in deciding to do whatever it is I'm fearful about. There's nothing quite like the joy and growth in it, feeling fabulous and fearless.

I've had more courage than I ever thought possible in choosing courage over fear. And that has allowed endless possibilities now and for the future.

Hold them close in your heart

Each time I lost a parent my heart shattered. I felt deeply the depth of love I had for each of them. Preserving in my heart, their unconditional love, support and age-old wisdom, that I used to so often let ride over me, an irreplaceable hole is now filled with beautiful unforgettable memories. How to move on without them?

My parents loved being by the sea and now I'm fortunate to live by the sea, I think of them often as I walk the beach and cliff tops. I sit and watch the ebb and flow of the waves on the shore and wonder what life is like for them in heaven. I still talk to them often, ask their advice and wait for answers. I look for signs, there are always signs, you just know when you know!

It's been so difficult to let them go and carry on without them but I've realised that our time on earth is a precious gift. Life is vibrant, full of amazing opportunities, experiences and beautiful moments to embrace. We must continue our own journey, as they would have wished.

And if you're lucky enough to still have your parents around, embrace their love, listen to their wisdom and hold them close in your heart.

Let your inner Goddess ROAR

Reading the poem 'Too much woman' by Ev Yan Witney, a knot gripped my stomach and tears flowed. The words cut through me like a knife. Many of those words were said to me. They were untrue. I felt judged and hurt. Their innocence and non-understanding minds could not comprehend my courage to allow the awakening goddess in me to be seen.

It was not my ego or self-centredness but an eagerness to express myself, my growth and my experiences for the benefit of all. In my early years I would give too much of me to others. I would lose myself and follow conditioned society, until eventually, through my deep dive into yoga, I found the courage to break free and find myself.

In my early fifties, my healing path of self-enquiry and self-love began. It took a great amount of strength and courage to confront my traumas and fears, to begin the healing process of 'letting go' and applying self love, allowing myself to be seen. When we heal and show ourselves, this ripples out into the world to help and allow others to heal and be seen. Don't allow anyone to bruise your inner Goddess, do not feel you have to hide away.

You are more than enough and worthy of showing your true beautiful self. Find your inner strength and courage and let your inner Goddess ROAR unapologetically.

Surrendering to the Moon's wisdom, she knows

Lodging at a friend's house during lockdown, putting myself back together after a broken marriage. 'What next?' was my question. I had no idea. I felt like 'surrendering' was the only thing left to do.

At first, it felt completely like just giving up but I had a sense that I didn't have to make a decision. I just needed to trust the universe to present me the right path.

I prayed that evening to the new moon for direction. The next morning, as I awoke, like magic, it came as the first thought in my head. 'Apply for a job in Cornwall'. I'd set that seed some seven years previously.

Cornwall had been my dream place to live. It had filled me with joy every time I visited and tears when I'd left. Three hundred miles away though, it meant starting again, leaving my children, family, lifelong friends and my business.

I trusted the divine; the fear was there but so was the excitement; I was flooded with so many emotions, I embraced them all. Inside I found enormous courage and strength. Life wasn't easy at first living in Cornwall, I'd given up so much to be there but this beautiful county filled my heart with joy. Two years on, I feel blessed to be living the dream. I've grown as a person and still work with moon and revel in her wisdom. Whatever you're going through, ask the moon, she knows.

As a mother to a son, Farideh has consistently asserted herself and stood up for her child.

She's found her voice in many roles - as a mother, daughter, sister, business owner and partner.

"Love," she emphasises, "serves as the foundation for advocating for oneself effectively." She believes that as one fosters inner peace, the need for self-advocacy diminishes, becoming increasingly superfluous.

Farideh chose to pen her chapter with a particular audience in mind: you. Her keen awareness of the heart's journey and its capacity to forge connections with others inspired her decision.

@faridehfotografie

FARIDEH DIEHL

Becoming a mother brings so much more than a child

Birth and death. Allies in the game of life. Like yin and yang, they're both aspects of a whole. The soul of my beloved grandmother said goodbye shortly before that of my son Vincent manifested in this dimension. She gave me the experience of a giving, nurturing love, which I could now pass on to my son.

However, with the birth of him, my own inner child also awakened and demanded attention to be seen and embraced. The projected story of a 'healed' world collided with the unseen story of an inner world that was not healed at all!

My greatest wish was and still is, to avoid unknowingly burdening my child with my baggage! My wish is to weave wings of light and love for him instead. My desire for authenticity meant I needed to leave my marriage though. I've thought about it so many times, at no time did I see this as a 'failure' but I did feel the sadness of my own deception that led me into the marriage in the first place.

In the deepest shadows, one finds the brightest treasures. The gift of being a mother, experiencing this all-encompassing love, simultaneously enabled me to recognise my own inner child. Never had I felt life's emotional highs and lows so intensely!

My heart jumps for joy with gratitude for the gifts another life brought me. Becoming a mother gave me the gift of gratitude for it all.

Constant change and a sense of allowing is my secret

At fifty-seven years old, after living my entire life in Germany, I took on a radical change. I sold almost all of my belongings and gave up my photo studio. I packed up my car and headed off to live in Mallorca.

With the open-hearted and like-minded people, as well as its geographical proximity, I shifted from the known to the unknown, full of new possibilities.

Since then, constant change and a sense of allowing for the unexpected have become my trusted companions. Throughout this journey of change, the interplay of magic and tragedy have both amazed and confused my mind. I feel I've been forced into reinventing my self-conception and with it, the way I encounter life.

This change has been spiritual and therapeutic work. The people who accompanied me on that journey have given me the strength and confidence to allow me to write a new story for myself, the end of which is open.

So here I am, with all my new understanding, still laden with ignorance. I'm still challenged to face my fears and at the same time, surrender to my dreams and visions.

If you find yourself reading my words on this page, I invite you to...believe the unexplainable, surrender to the unknown and accept the limitations. And with that, be ready to be surprised by the unexpected and most of all...be here and now. Those, I believe, are the ingredients for the recipe of 'change'.

FINDING THE DEFINITION OF SUCCESS FOR YOU

My professional career path developed from my passions. I've always loved working with people, being creative in influencing a design process and having a rhythm that grounds me, while allowing me the flexibility to respond spontaneously to changes.

These parameters resulted in my self-employment as an agency owner and photographer. However, after over thirty-five 'successful' years, I'm faced with the question of how success is actually defined for me. My understanding of success has changed significantly since I began. My intention to show the beauty, in the essence of people and things, is unbroken. But today, it is the flaws and inconsistencies I see that make me aware that 'perfection' arises from an interplay. If you trust in yourself through the flow of seemingly conflicting elements (of life), you allow movement to arise, out of its integration. This leads to a consistency, which then again reveals a rhythm that nourishes the flow itself.

So, the interplay of seemingly conflicting elements become tangible with the tension they create. Consistency is thus created by letting go of the longing for it. Success to me, is entering the dancefloor of life by embracing the various roles, being as much the choreographer as the student, the designer as well as the receiver. It's an interplay of 'giving in' and 'trusting', much like the lead and follow in dance. All the 'faulty' steps are part of the learning process - welcome them gracefully with a laugh and move on.

It's about not fearing the unknown and keeping your heart and senses open for possibilities. This attitude will generate synchronicities that will nourish (or deepen) your trust in the flow of life.

MOVE TOWARDS YOUR TRUTH

It sometimes takes a whole life to find one's own truth. My truth started emerging when I no longer wanted to fit the map that my culture and country of origin had given me. I became aware of being 'out of tune' with the values, habits, rituals and conditions that had determined my life until that point. And I had to trust my inner voice and give it prerogative over reason and doubt, which gave me the strength to end all material ties with my homeland Germany. I packed my belongings into my car and drove off to discover a new unknown country.

My life is no less challenging since then, in fact, rather the opposite but I feel the coherence of my decision confirmed every single day - inside and out.

I believe you have to be willing to take whatever life presents to you - every experience and every encounter. Practice loving more, to become more compassionate and to keep an open heart. All polarities, I find, are fragments of one and the same truth...everything is connected. The deception of our perception, always lies in our limited ability to be able to use our senses. For instance, white light contains all the colours of the visible light spectrum. When you mix Cyan, Magenta and Yellow you get Black. Both 'non-colours' are the origin or consequence of a mixture of colours.

Life includes all possibilities; don't be deceived by the limitations of our perceptiveness. Trust your own path and intuition. They will lead you towards your unique truth.

STEPPING OUT OF SILENT, UNCONSCIOUS PARTICIPATION AGREEMENTS

We are the story we tell ourselves....but where does that story come from? I've often wondered, did I write this role myself? Or was it a mosaic of desires, fears, hopes and expectations projected onto me?

My longing for answers and my fear of 'imploding emotionally', led me to therapy. For over five years, I explored my shadows and I've been able to say goodbye to, to accept and peacefully conclude my 'yesterday', in order to be able to live today.

To face my shadows and limitations, to experience compassion and forgiveness meant I could embrace myself. This wild, dark, painful but infinitely healing and peace-creating journey to the origins of my Self, gave me inner trust.

It gave me the strength to accept that I couldn't heal all the open wounds and I had to let go of my longing to be seen, embracing my flaws and the flaws of others.

I had to acknowledge 'imperfection' and trust that love always heals in its own mysterious ways. The map of self-knowledge leads us into unknown territory. It's worth being courageous and trusting ourselves into uncertainty. Our stories can be rewritten.

THE GOAL IS THE JOURNEY

My transformative journey began with a profound heartfelt question. As I travelled through India, exploring the various languages of Yoga, I heard 'Who am I?'.

I considered myself a conscious individual but soon realised I'd fed my mind with knowledge and techniques designed to avoid pain and ignorance. The illusion of control I had did nothing to stop the darkness within me growing. It became increasingly challenging to access the light and ease I craved.

Fortunately, an encounter with an enlightened soul touched my heart and silenced my mind, allowing me to connect with my true essence and access the origins of my being. This newfound connection with my soul was a crucial step towards self-acceptance. I don't tend to follow teachings devotedly but I do preserve my curiosity. We're all teachers and students and they can be helpful companions in times of change and uncertainty. It requires trust to reveal one's own vulnerability and explore the answers within.

Allow yourself to doubt and question your truth. Be open to advice and to repeatedly forgive yourself and others for the adversities of your journey. The goal isn't to find the answer, whether true or false, the goal is the journey itself, towards inner peace and love.

THE HEART MUST BREAK SO YOU LEARN TO TRUST IT FULLY

It's 1993, I'm in New York. I was almost eighteen and with my head full of images and my heart wide open, I stormed into a life experience with naivety and a thirst for adventure!

With little more than dreams and curiosity in my luggage, I placed myself in the dependency of the man who was the reason for this journey.

A babysitting job allowed me one hot meal a day and paid my dance school bills. We lived with little, made new friends every day, shared a shower with eight people and froze in winter. We'd sit on the steps to our house in summer, enjoying the colourful wild life that passed by. It was a wondrous yet cruel time. New inspirations went hand-in-hand with the dying of illusions of security and trust. I was desperate and happy at the same time; I lost who I thought I was.

But I gained great gifts in rediscovering myself and trusting the unexpected! I let go of naive images of romantic love and embraced my joy in dancing. I now realise my heart had to break so I could trust it truly. Love isn't an idea, it's lived joy that lives in you!

The injuries and scars are necessary: they wake us up to the unseen, the repressed and the ignorant – they are our blessing.

THE TIME OF THE LONE WOLF IS OVER

Life is but a circle, an eternal dance of atoms, a vibration of infinite frequencies and I am a pigment of the colour palette. I am a hair blowing in the breeze and a sigh of light and shadow. We are all stones in the constantly changing mosaic composition of the inexplicable...and...we all need each other.

Looking back, it seems that I've had to stand up for myself alone. I have 'stood my ground'. And now I feel the need to collaborate with likeminded women.

We mature women often share the personal experiences and insights of our individual pasts but more than that, we are called upon to face the challenges of the present together...with the authenticity and knowledge we've each gained.

We inspire, provoke, support, embrace and empower each other, in the constant process of change and growth. We share our sincerity, face impermanence with dignity and respect and we are an example for the next generation.

I believe, we're experiencing a time of massive external transformation. Existing rules are being questioned and new paradigms are being pushed. Mastering these shifts on a personal as well as a social level, requires a willingness to connect to each other, to enter into co-operations, to cultivate exchanges and 'connectedness'.

The time of the lone wolf is over. This wonderful joint book project, is therefore for me, a model and synonym for my personal inner readiness to peel myself out of the comfort of the familiar and to dive into the flow of the unknown. It's also an invitation to trust the support and important exchange of my female travel companions.

We are many, dear sister. We are one.

Cathy, a mother and a grandmother, found her biggest inspiration in her own mother when it came to finding and using her voice.

Even as a child, she wielded her voice to stand up to a domineering father, asserting her identity as a woman. In her early twenties, she tackled the rampant alcoholism that ran in the female line of her family.

Throughout her career, she asserted her voice with clarity and strength, navigating the predominantly male world of advertising.

Deeply inspired by the power of women, Cathy hopes to empower you with her story and her journey of overcoming her battles.

CATHY McPHERSON

A LETTER TO MY ADDICTION

I got sober at twenty-three years of age, after becoming addicted to alcohol. I was advised to write a letter to my addiction to help me face up to how dependent I had become. This is the letter I wrote, all those years ago.

Dear Alcohol

I can appreciate how much you helped me in my early years of drinking. I always felt less than and was very over sensitive, I had no self-esteem. You made me feel invisible.

I could be fun and free from my obsession of Self, I felt attractive and vibrant. We had some great times together. Somewhere along the way, it became harder to reach the high you once gave me. I would need to drink more of you, in different ways, at different times to try and get the elation you once gave me. You seemed to become more elusive and you made me feel so ill the next day that sometimes I couldn't function.

I can now see how I became dependent on you, I couldn't go a day without needing you and the drinks started earlier, even though I was constantly letting people down and not turning up to work, feeling like shit. I still managed to pour you down my neck until I passed out. You were no fun anymore. I was depressed, lonely and unpopular and everyone hated me. But most of all, I hated myself.

Once I realised and surrendered to the fact that you were now destroying me, I decided to part company and one day at a time, I stay away from you. I respect that you are always there waiting for me but today, I choose not to pour you down my neck. I have a great life now and have had for the last thirty-four years.

May you rest in peace.

Catherine

ACCEPT WHO YOU ARE

From very young, I always wanted long hair. Cursed with fine, fragile hair that broke even on silk pillow cases, my mum kept my hair really short. A hairdresser told her that would help thicken it up. It didn't. And I came to hate my hair. Always feeling like a boy, I envied the girls with their ponytails and thick hair!

By age ten, I would put silk scarves on my head imagining what it would be like to have feminine, beautiful locks. I spent my adult life chasing the dream of long hair...extensions, wigs, vitamin tablets! I visited trichologists to grow it, despite it snapping off at my shoulders! I'd constantly compare myself to other women, telling myself I was ugly and unattractive to men who preferred long hair.

It was a friend of mine, who said how cool I looked with short hair! She said I stood out from the crowd and that she was jealous, that my small pixie face was made for short hair!

'To constantly compare, is to constantly despair', she said and that was my light bulb moment! This short-haired girl has come a long way...I've been blonde, platinum, black, red and orange, sometimes all together! Please love ALL of you. It's such a wasted time comparing yourself to others. Be unique and beautiful, you're a child of the universe.

FIND OUT THE ROOT CAUSE

At school, I found it so hard to concentrate and remember anything. I tried hard to pay attention but my foot would tap or my muscles would twitch, my eyes would water. I couldn't focus, I was bored, my teachers voice was grating. The words on the blackboard danced and this would be in a lesson I enjoyed!

Exams were the worst, I tried to revise but would read pages of books and not remember a thing. I'd write notes but given how haphazard they were, I couldn't read them the next day.

The rest of my family are high achievers. Very bright, they thought I was thick, as did my teachers. 'Below average', they said and I felt below average. It affected my self-esteem.

I didn't go to University (obviously) but through luck more than design, I found myself working in advertising, an industry that relies on personality, creativity and communication.

I loved it from day one. I was fifty before my employer suggested I have a dyslexia test. I'd been at board level for twenty-five years, so I knew I wasn't thick but I still struggled with writing and reading, I'd just hidden it. I was diagnosed dyslexic! Not in all areas but a lot. I'd compensated so well but that had been exhausting.

If you feel mis-wired, my advice is to get tested, it could make your life much easier!

ARTICULATE YOURSELF

I've always been fiery and quick to temper. Guilty of repressing my truth and feelings, I can explode and be quite hurtful with my words.

An example would be if my husband isn't spending enough time with me, I might be feeling de-prioritised (because of his work or his time riding motorbikes with his friends). I want to be understanding, patient and thoughtful, so I don't say anything, I try and 'fake it to make it' and don't complain.

But resentment builds, I narrate a conversation in my head which sounds reasonable, then when I speak, it comes out all wrong and I create an argument, shouting and being very judgemental.

This causes further rifts and I push him away more. However, I learnt on a course to sit down at least once a week and follow the PIES model. Each partner speaks without interruption...saying how they feel, 'Physically', 'Intellectually', 'Emotionally' and 'Spiritually'.

This has saved my marriage many times. It's allowed me to say how I feel without being aggressive or accusatory. It also gave me insight into my husband who hadn't been one for sharing his feelings either. Both of us must stick to using 'I' statements and avoid using 'you'. My husband is more in touch with his feelings and articulates them in a way he's never been able to before, it's a great model for honest communication.

JUMPING SHIP TO SELF-EMPLOYMENT

Do it! I wanted to make enough money to last me twelve months before I jumped. I was aware of the importance of sales and marketing, I knew I'd have to sell my services, so I made sure I was comfortable doing that. I felt confident that my career in advertising stood me in good stead, marketing and promotion were second nature to me. I was always ambitious, surrounded by inspirational, talented and great teachers. As a result, I did really well and learnt a lot about running companies. After fifteen years, I became restless, I knew enough about myself to know I enjoyed constant change and would embrace a challenge!

I took on freelance consultant roles, working with agencies who couldn't afford full-time resources but needed help in specific areas.

This worked for me, some contracts were two weeks, some six months, either way, each opportunity taught me a lot and soon my skill set became very broad and I could turn my hand to most areas of business.

Making this move was the best thing I've ever done, my drive ensured I was never without work and eventually my husband pointed out to me that I was undercharging. I did some research and it seemed I was indeed selling myself short. I tripled my daily rate immediately and the first time I put a quote in, the agency didn't bat an eyelid and they signed it off straight away.

I couldn't believe it. If you, like me, want to be in control of your own destiny and play to your strengths, passions and be paid your worth, then I highly recommend taking the jump.

FILL YOUR LIFE WITH PEOPLE YOU LOVE

Nobody ever tells you how to deal with grief. It's personal and one size doesn't fit all. I was fifty-five before I experienced real grief so I feel lucky, I hadn't lost anyone close to me before that. My parents were reaching a grand age of eighty-nine and ninety-five, so I had them around me a long time. Like all families, we had our ups and downs, life wasn't always rosy but when I finally got the call that Mum had days to live, I remember spending the last few precious days with her.

The lesson I learned is that nothing mattered other than the pure love I had for her and I really did. All hurt of the past was evaporated and I just kept telling her how much I loved her over and over again.

On her passing, there was a massive hole in my life which I'm still learning to fill. My advice would be to fill your life with people you love, don't waste time on people not worthy of your love. Receiving and giving love is precious.

STEP UP FOR YOURSELF

As a young woman I always wanted to be looked after by a man. As a child, I often felt lonely and neglected. Unconscious bias was evident in my home from the age of four, when my father sent my two elder brothers to boarding school (aged seven) and I was kept home.

A very successful Urologist, he worked a lot, which provided us a very privileged lifestyle, however, the emotional and physical contact was missing. He was very tough, remote and never once told me he loved me. I never had intimate conversations with him. Lost and alone, from my teenage years through to my forties, I searched for a man, who would look after me financially and emotionally, someone who'd be there, whatever happened. But I picked men who were capable of neither.

Many broken relationships, heartache and disappointment later, a therapist told me I needed to step up and be financially and emotionally there for myself! Encouraged to leave the injured child behind me and step into my power, slowly I became financially successful, learning to be my own therapist, friend and wise woman.

Only then, did I meet a man equal to me, who was able to give me unconditional love and support in a healthy way. Twenty years on, I love and am very grateful to my husband Ian for showing up when I stepped up for myself.

VISUALISE YOUR DREAMS

I was familiar with mood boards. In advertising, we often saw the creative team put them together for campaigns. They explained to clients what their delivery would look like using imagery, tone of voice, genre, font and general look and feel.

When I qualified as a coach, my teacher empowered us to put together our own mood boards. You either print pictures from the internet or cut pictures from magazines and stick them onto card to create the future you want.

Mine included lots of schnauzer dogs (my passion), a beautiful modern house in the country, a home abroad, holidays to exotic places, retiring at fifty-five, using my coaching degree to deliver training (image of a class room) and family images of social occasions. I had no idea how I was going to achieve any of this but I diligently put my board up in my office and looked at it every day, giving my dream to the universe and remaining open that one day I could realise this dream.

Today, I write this with two schnauzers looking at me! I'm in rented accommodation whilst my husband builds our dream home, I'm off to Spain to stay at our apartment next month and I'm semi-retired!

The journey here just happened naturally. I'm amazed at how it happened. I'm doing another mood board for the next few years. I really recommend you do this as a gift to your dreams.

Jackie is part of an all-female, women-led Mastermind group. This collective of wonderful women, along with her close female friends, have inspired her to use her voice authentically, expressing her personal thoughts rather than just echoing the views of others.

Her voice gains its most potent strength in the workplace. Navigating male-dominated environments, she has had to articulate her ideas with clarity and conviction. She has expanded her vocal expressions in numerous ways —from singing in a choir to contributing to this book.

She hopes that her words will comfort and embolden other women, reassuring them that they are not alone and that they have the strength and courage to face any situation life presents.

JACKIE CLIFFORD

Don't compare yourself to others, celebrate your own achievements

I learned a new word when I started working on myself and my business – it's called 'comparisonitis'. For years, I thought I needed extra qualifications, more experience, greater achievements or expertise to be really valid in my work. But as I started to confide in others about how I felt, mainly the women in my life, I realised so many of us were having similar conversations with the voices in our heads.

We used the word 'comparisonitis' to describe that feeling of always comparing ourselves to another, their version being better than our version of us.

That comparison conversation in my head is sometimes quiet, barely there but sometimes loud. It can actually feel like quite a motivator on occasion but often, in reality, it's just damaging. In the past when I've looked at someone else's seemingly fabulous life, I seemed to decide that mine measured up less favourably.

I had an experience a few years ago where I was listening to a wonderful woman sharing her inspirational story and all I could think, was how she'd had more advantages than me, that she was probably born to achieve and that life could never be mine.

The impact that had on me was despair and desperation. I couldn't celebrate her with the joy her story deserved! I try these days not to compare my journey with others, I try to hear their stories and learn from them with an open heart and mind.

My advice to you is this; if you can learn not to compare your journey with others, you'll hear the possibility in their story and be able to map that possibility onto your own life, with an open heart and mind. I find that when I do this now, I feel so much better...I'm able to celebrate their achievements and acknowledge my own.

You have important things to say!

I'm passing through my fifties and I'm learning that it's ok to put my voice, opinions and words out there into the world. For so long, I believed that others had more to say than me, I masked my light behind those I perceived to be burning more brightly.

I was brought up with the 'children should be seen and not heard'/'don't speak until you're spoken to' era. It's only now that I'm realising the damaging impact of those messages.

I had rather a loud voice as a child, mainly when I was talking to my Great Grandmother (who was deaf) but I read very well too, so I was often chosen to read aloud from the pulpit in Church.

I felt ok with that, I was reading someone else's words, I wasn't expressing my own opinion. That theme continued through my work, sharing more of other people's words, ideas and voices rather than my own. I'm noticing now that I'm putting up my thoughts too, I'm sharing them more readily and my ideas are being offered up for consideration.

Your voice, dear reader, is as valuable as any other on the planet. Be visible, it's perfectly wonderful to speak before someone invites you to do so!

You can handle whatever life throws at you!

It was a dark and rainy night, I was driving back from a weekend of work with my colleague. All of a sudden, we heard and felt something really weird happening to my Vauxhall Nova! We were on the M1 (the multi-lane motorway linking London to the north of England) with cars and lorries speeding past us as we pulled up onto the hard shoulder.

My fear was confirmed, we had a flat tyre! I found the spare wheel and the jack, found the jacking point and raised the car from the ground, so that I could release the wheel nuts. Once that was done, I pumped the jack so the car was in the air and I changed the wheel. I did that! I just got on and did it!

I use this memory to help me remember that, when the proverbial shit hits the fan, I can deal with it. I got us back on the road, home, safe and sound – all on my own!

My lesson: whatever life throws at you, you can – and you will – handle it. Dear reader, if there's one thing I would want you to hear in this story, it's this: you can handle whatever life throws at you!

You have all the resources you need and they will just appear, right when you need them. Trust in you – you are amazing!

Someone else's opinion of you is not actually you!

When I was at primary school, I remember preparing for some sort of assembly or concert. My class was singing and the teacher told some of us (including me) that we weren't allowed to sing out loud...we should mime...apparently, we were 'growlers'!

From that day on, I believed I couldn't sing. And I didn't. Maybe in the car or bath but I'd never have let anyone actually hear me! Fast forward forty years and my Mum discovered a local community choir called Funky Voices. I don't know what made me do it but I went with her to a taster session and I've been a member of the choir for years now. No audition, no judgement, just the chance to sing with others.

My voice is part of something now and it gets bigger every time we rehearse or do a gig, I've even signed up to sing at the Edinburgh Festival this year!

If you're hearing someone else's voice in your head, sharing their beliefs about you, ask yourself... 'Is there is any hard evidence for what they're saying?'. They saw you in 'one moment' in time, they shared (maybe without your permission) the only thing that they were able to see - through their own clouded and coloured lens of the world.

Take a look in the mirror and see yourself as the person you know you are!

It's not personal....

I grew up in a town in Essex in the UK. I went to primary school in the 1970s, the daughter of an English mother and an Indian father who left when I was a toddler, I grew up in what I now see as 'a room without mirrors'.

What I mean by that, is I didn't see myself as others saw me. To me, I just saw 'Jackie' but to my classmates and teachers, I was the only brown child in the entire school! I was different and as a result, I experienced some teasing and comments that made me feel separate and lonely. Of course, I took them to heart, I spent years thinking those comments were all about me!

Now I'm only just realising that those comments weren't personal to me at all. Their comments were judgements based on what they had heard from others! Nothing more.

Know that deep in your heart and be kinder to yourself, more forgiving of others - they don't know, what they don't know. Shine brightly - it's not personal!

DON'T PUSH SOMEONE, LET THEM FIGURE IT OUT

I grew up surrounded by amazing, strong women. We were a household of four generations. the eldest of which was my Great Grandmother, born in 1878. My childhood was filled with stories of her life as a woman in service, in London, during the reign of Queen Victoria!

My life (and thinking) has been shaped by these incredible women. One of the things I will eternally be grateful for is the fact that they never pushed me or put pressure on me. Instead, I knew they always just wanted me to be safe, well and happy.

I don't have children. If I did, I would hope that I'd role-model this. I was never pressured by my mother or any of the other women in my life, to be or do anything specific.

I remember being encouraged and nudged. I remember my mother respecting me when I wasn't ready to step outside my comfort zone; in fact, she climbed more trees than I ever did when we were out with my friends!

By being allowed to go at my own pace, I was able to find my own rhythm. I never felt resentment for being made to do something that didn't feel right, I was able to develop my own set of values and principles to live by.

Go gently with those around you. Don't place pressure on them. It's ok to give someone a nudge sometimes but don't push them – unless someone specifically asks for a push and even then, find out what they actually really need, the chances are they can figure out what they really need without too much interference.

BEING SAFE CAN BE TOO RESTRICTING

As I've started to look back on my life so far and question why I made certain decisions, I realise that a massive amount of my self-talk was about keeping me safe and not being hurt.

I've never been very 'physically' intelligent, I've never used my body much for sports or physical activity, I've been too busy protecting myself! I'm not quite sure what I thought would happen to me if I broke a bone or tore a tendon, I've never had the chance to find out but in recent years I've pushed against that.

A decade ago, I did the London Moonwalk (a walking overnight marathon), it was gruelling and it took forever but I did it with three of my friends, including my Mum who was just approaching her seventieth birthday. In more recent times, I've tried HIIT training in the gym, yoga, pilates and I've discovered that walking in nature is great exercise for the mind and spirit as well as the body.

I understand the importance of exploring the whole person now...the mental, spiritual, emotional and physical sides of us. Even if physical intelligence isn't where I personally excel, my body still deserves to be used in different ways.

Being too safe can be truly restricting. In future, I'll continue to do my risk assessments but I've quietened the voice that tells me I'm not good at physical things and just do the things that bring me joy!

CARRY ON LEARNING ABOUT YOURSELF, YOU'RE DOING REALLY WELL

My life is and always has been about learning. I believe the day we stop learning, is the day they should be nailing the lid on the box!

I've learned so much and yet sometimes I feel like it's taking so much time to really learn; especially about my own personal patterns of behaviour, patterns I keep repeating but would love to change. They seem so ingrained, they come round again and again, like a groove on an outdated vinyl album.

I notice that certain words or tones of voice take me straight back into old patterns. If I hear 'you're a drama queen' for instance or a criticism about why I've done something a certain way, I leap into defence, either retreating into myself or bursting out fighting.

Neither of those are helpful and they certainly don't help my relationships. I'm slowly learning to forgive myself for those knee-jerk reactions.

I notice and celebrate times when I react as I'd want, rather than the way my physiology and triggers dictate. I take a breath and a step back. Sometimes I walk away altogether.

Sometimes difficult situations aren't of your making, they're about where other people are. You're not responsible for everyone and everything. Learn about yourself and your patterns, in your own time, you're doing perfectly ok.

Toni's childhood set her up to understand the power of the bully and the strength it takes to stand your ground.

She has stood her ground in so many ways, especially during her corporate career. She remembers using her voice most prominently when she refused to make thousands of people redundant – she left herself instead and started her own business.

Her early mentor John Donnelly was a great support to her and privately, her husband Richard is always there for her.

She wrote her stories to be able to give back, believing that if she impacted just one woman positively, it was more than worth doing!
Her journey embodies resilience, compassion and empowerment.

@tonieastwoodcoach

TONI EASTWOOD OBE, MBA

CONFIDENCE COMES FROM FACING YOUR FEARS

I've struggled with confidence most of my life. I vividly remember at twenty-two desperately wanting to be successful, having monthly performance meetings with my boss. He'd tell me I had potential, which I never believed!

I dreaded those meetings, I literally could not speak about myself, I'd start and just want to cry, I knew what I wanted to say but a lump in my throat meant I wouldn't say anything. I remember the meeting that flipped the switch though. He was fed up and to be honest, so was I, with myself. "Toni this is pointless" he said, "you don't give me anything, it's just one way, do you want this?". I was devastated, "YES I DO" I said, very clearly, trying to make my body language match just how much I wanted it.

That was that, he set me monthly challenges. The more I did, the better I became. I now know, that confidence comes from facing fears head on and getting into action. I am so grateful for his belief in me. I use my voice now to stand out and to give back.

You don't need a mentor though, think about how you can set yourself little challenges that allow you to face into your fears, perhaps a weekly or monthly goal that will stretch you beyond your comfort zone and gradually build the trust in yourself, that you can do this.

If you have a friend to share your plans with, you'll have some accountability and someone to share your success with.

Every time you achieve a challenge, give yourself a high five and say "that's like me!". If you can do that in the mirror, there's only one result, your smile will beam back at you.

SCHEDULING CAN GIVE GREAT STRUCTURE

Thirty years ago, I started out on a quest to find the secrets to success.

Mostly driven by my desire to squash my own demons, I researched everything I could and developed a model that worked for me.

It's very practical. I needed structure, I call it 'time blocking'. I block my day into ninety-minute slots. This is my schedule based on this;

• 6 – 7.30am is all about me (meditation and exercise)

• 9 – 11.30am is all about creation (I get clear about my goals and assess what needs my focus)

• 2.00 – 3.30pm for me is all about sales in my business (I work on whatever needs to be done, follow-up calls, emails, preparing leaflets). I also use the acronym W.I.N. (What's Important Now) to help me decide how to use this slot.

In between my ninety-minute slots, I do something that's doesn't need my brain power. I get some movement in or have lunch, check in with my colleagues. My colleagues laugh when they catch me doing star jumps or burpees in the office, it's important for me not to sit down all day!

• My evening slot is about time with my hubby, to cook and eat properly.

• Finally, my 8-9.30pm slot is back to me (journalling, a good book, winding down)

Structuring my days like this has been super powerful for me, a real game changer.

CHOOSE COURAGE AND VULNERABILITY, OVER COMFORT

If there's one tip, I really wished I'd been given a long time ago, it would be...'let go and put yourself out there, even if you can't choose the outcome'. I probably was given that tip but maybe I wasn't ready to hear it, I certainly wasn't ready to be courageous or vulnerable.

The demons I've fought through life so far though have made me quite courageous, I'd go as far as to say they've been a virtue and I have always been tenacious. But...and it's a big 'but', the fear of being vulnerable, of really showing who I am, of really going after what I really want, has held me back. I was frightened what others may think.

At forty-four, I decided to step forward into growth, rather than back into safety and everything changed for me. I set up the business that I'd been dreaming about for ten years, at fifty-one, I wrote the book I knew was inside me and at fifty-three, I started delivering my own programme – the one I wrote eight years before and paid someone else to deliver!

I choose growth. I choose courage. I choose vulnerability. I choose courage over comfort; I choose vulnerability and I put myself out there.

I show up now and take action even if it scares the shit out of me. I'm prepared to have a go at something I care about, even if I might fail. I choose to expose myself emotionally even if I might cry in public. To show up and be seen when I can't control the outcome, that's what courage and vulnerability looks like for me now.

Don't get to the end of your life asking 'What if?'. Take one tiny little step forward into growth today, then take a tiny step tomorrow. Next day and the next are compound effects and that is infinite. Step into your infinite potential, you've got this!

OPTIMISE YOUR ENERGY

I can often find myself procrastinating or needing to find extra willpower to get me going. I used to just try and plough through until I found this equation...

$$\text{Motivation} = \text{Value} \times \text{Expectancy} / \text{Impulsivity} \times \text{Delay}$$

In other words, motivation equals 'how fired up I am about getting something' (the value) and how confident I am that I can have it (expectancy). When I really want something and I really know I can get it, I'm more likely to show up and work hard. When I'm feeling demotivated, or stuck, I run the numbers. Out of ten, how motivated am I? How fired up am I? and How confident am I that I can have it?

When I've done that, I need to make sure I'm not distracted by screen notifications (Impulsivity) and that helps me focus on the micro goals in front of me, so I'm always making progress (Delay).

I have found this strategy super powerful. I've also realised there's an even more powerful piece to add into the mix though...energy.

$$\text{Motivation} = \text{ENERGY} \times (\text{Value} \times \text{Expectancy} / \text{Impulsivity} \times \text{Delay})$$

If my energy sucks, the whole equation falls apart. When I'm tired, I just don't see the world the same way. Optimise your energy, always optimise your energy.

OBSTACLES WILL ALWAYS MAKE YOU STRONGER

I've never shared this, part of me doesn't want to but a bigger part knows that if this story can help just one person, then I absolutely should share it.

A few years ago, I was excited that my book 'The Woman Beyond' was finished and was being delivered the next week. I'd spent the summer writing it.

I was proud and a little worried. Sharing my story for the first time felt very raw. Then I took a phone call. My business was to be inspected the following week. I can't deny I was nervous. The next week came and for a whole week, five inspectors sifted through my business. They put us through the wringer and grilled all my staff.

Despite excellent client feedback, it seemed they had already made their decision. Sat alone in my office, I kept my grace and remained calm but on the inside, I was so angry, their decision was going to kill my business overnight.

I burst into tears, devastated. Such an incredulous difference to the joy I'd felt a few days before about my book...that was the day the first print run of books arrived too. I felt like, in their one ridiculous decision, they had taken my business and my moment of celebration and trashed it! I spent the weekend rethinking what I wanted, both in business and in life.

I ended up realigning everything with a much stronger purpose. That purpose was about service, a tight team and surrounding myself with people who shared my values and my vision. I had to let half my team go but we started anew. I used my anger and this devastating event as fuel for growth.

My mantra is 'OMMS' – Obstacles Make Me Stronger – they really do.

BRING IT ON, YOU'LL TRUST YOURSELF!

One thing I know in life, is that it's not an easy ride, no matter how much we'd all like it to be. From the age of five, a petite, brown curly haired, small innocent little girl, I had to pretend to be fearless.

Bullies would lay in wait and taunt my name - it was a boys name. They'd pick on my clothes, because my Mum made them (which I loved!). At seven, I'd run as fast as I could to get the hell out, before they'd catch me. I'd run across the hall. out the doors to the gates, where my Mum's friend collected her kids. I knew then, I could walk home safely and ignore the name calling. It didn't end there, in senior school I'd hide in doorways and sit in the classroom for safety. I never told anyone, my parents never knew, until they started appearing at my front door, threatening my siblings.

Even as I write this, I have tears running down my face, I am fifty-six for gods sake and this still hurts like hell but I can honestly say that after a lot of soul searching, I can thank them. I know I can face whatever comes and that's served me well!

In my career, especially the last twelve years in business when the shit really hit the fan, I knew I'd always get through. I will always get back up and I will always have confidence and tenacity, even if, now and again, I know I'm still faking it!

ATTITUDE OF GRATITUDE

I learned the hard way that what you think, is what you create! By my forties I had realised the profound effect of my own thinking, the not feeling 'good enough', the lack of confidence or the lack of money and how that was manifesting. I've been blown away many times by the power of 'flipping the switch', when we're able to recognise when we're in negative spirals of self-doubt or sabotage and then are able to flip the switch to a more positive angle. Choose to see the good and find the opportunity out of whatever's happening.

What you focus on develops and grows. A positive mindset and attitude means facing our challenges in an optimistic way and finding gratitude, even if it's just for the tiny things.

The number one most powerful solution I have personally put into my daily practice is a Daily Gratitude Shower – it's the practice of writing down just five things I'm most grateful for each day.

I've heard that scientists say that writing even just five things we're grateful for each week boosts our happiness by twenty-five percent! What's not to love!

SPEAK TO THE LITTLE GIRL YOU WERE

At fifty plus, I still have moments of fear that stop me in my tracks, I never liked myself, I can be standoffish too. It's a defence mechanism from being bullied at school. I've worked hard to try to be rid of this, I've done meditation, taking breaths to recalibrate, affirmations, I have a fucking armoury of those!

But I've realised that I left that little five-year-old girl in me alone. I ignored her feelings and ploughed on regardless. I took the tenacity she gave me and the drive that she built, yet I buried her and left in the dark. I realised I had to work with her, in order to help me. I consider her feelings now, I tell her I love her. She protected me then and she protects me now.

Every morning I ask her what she wants. When I started, she just folded her arms looked me up and down and told me to 'Fuck off!'. I didn't blame her.

I still told her I love her though and that I was there to listen.   Now when I ask her what she'd do in any situation, she gives it to me straight, tells me to toughen up, stop making excuses, to get over myself, whatever she thinks I need.

It's been so powerful for me. My guess is that your little girl is within you too, waiting to be heard and to be there for you. She has wise words, if not a few choice ones to start with!

Tap into her wisdom, she'll tell you what she thinks.

Speak to the little girl you were,
she has wise words for you

Inspired by a host of female leaders, Lenka Lutonska is her most recent influencer and guide.

A spaceholder for the divine feminine, Andrea is devoted to reclaiming a woman's birthright to gather and heal in sisterhood.

Her commitment to inspiring a broader community of women led her to write her chapter and she hopes her words help women find their flow, reconnect to themselves, trust their bodies and own their uniqueness.

@thewildwomanacademy

ANDREA JACKSON

WILD WOMAN AWAKE – DANCE WITH LIFE

I used to dance, always! I loved Soul and Motown...I just adored dancing. Somewhere along the way, I forgot. I loved yoga too but something else was calling. I came across tribal belly dance and I remembered!

Something woke up inside, my tribal roots were awakened and I began to dance again! There's something about giving ourselves the gift of freedom. When we give ourselves the permission to just let our bodies move, I found it helped elevate my mood and energy. Free dancing made me smile, I felt strong, sexy, feminine and confident in my body again.

Women must dance! We can all dance, it's like a sense of freedom for the soul. Music touched places in me that I hadn't even remembered, so going through the transition of menopause, adding dance really helped me move through grief and sadness. It helps me now celebrate all the great times too.

Music is so powerful and when we're dancing, our body can flow the energy through it, leaving us feeling uplifted and free.

You really can't get it wrong! Dance is a celebration of the female form, whatever age, size you are, it doesn't matter, it's an expression of you and it's so beautiful! Crank up the music and dance my love! You really will feel so much better!

MONEY IS FREEDOM

I never knew this, whoever tells you this? Money is freedom and it's choice! I never respected money or cared much about it either. I had always associated money with ego, so I resisted it like crazy!

Looking back, I always had enough though, no matter what, I was always ok. So now in my wisdom years I realise, I didn't need to worry about it as much as I did, that was such an energy drain!

I'm learning to make friends with money and see her as a beautiful source of energy that allows me both peace of mind and freedom. I'm learning to respect money and I've found a correlation between when I'm not respecting my personal energy, I find that the flow of abundance slows down. There seems to be a real connection there.

When I stop worrying and relax around money, my money flow increases. Always! When I recharge my energy, money flows again, every time! When I dismiss worrying thoughts about money, my money flow also increases and I feel free.

It feels so important for me to tell women to make a friend of money. I was never taught to save or invest, actually I was taught that making money was 'Men's work'. It feels to me now, as if women are really beginning to claim their place in the world of wealth and rightly so.

A mantra I've worked with, which I have found helpful in healing my own limiting mindset around money is...

"This is what a wealthy woman looks like"

When I began to repeat this mantra in the mirror daily, I felt so free and empowered. It changed my perception of what a wealthy woman could look like. It dawned on me that that woman could be me! And it can be you too. Try it, and see the magic unfold.

ALWAYS HAVE A RUNAWAY FUND

I never knew this, who tells you this kind of wisdom? I have come to know that money is independence, freedom and choice! I stayed in damaged relationships way longer than I needed to because I didn't have the money to leave. I didn't have that choice. It's so empowering to have an escape fund behind you.
I'm not saying you'll run away but it's always there, so you have the choice.

When you have your own bank account set up with a little fall-back money in it, it creates freedom and choice, it's like you can relax, you don't have to put up with or tolerate being bullied, controlled or treated badly. I've been stuck in tough situations, I know personally how it feels to be there, frustrated, controlled, powerless.

If you are this woman, reading this now, this could be a way out. Even if you can start saving just a few pounds a month, create the fund, even if it's in secret, set up the bank account. It's so empowering to see your little escape fund growing. A plan can begin to form and you can start dreaming about a life outside of this.
You just never know when you might need it.

JOURNAL...IT'S LIKE POLISHING A STEAMY MIRROR AFTER A SHOWER!

I love taking time to light a candle, sit with my Cacao, my journal and my heart. It gives me the opportunity to be fully present. I take life soooo seriously sometimes!

I push and I strive but I ask myself sometimes, what for? What if I chose to live in my flow, in the love lane, with my wisdom, love, joy and fun? It' a great big YES in my heart.

As I get older and wiser, the only thing I strive for, is a life that's uncomplicated. I simply follow what makes me happy, that's the real goal of life for me now. I've found that journaling really supports me, it unblocks me and creates more flow. Sitting in the quiet, listening to what's swooshing around in my head, letting the words fall onto the journal, it's like polishing the steamy mirror after my shower so I can see myself clearly again!

Something wonderful is sheltered inside of all of us. I know this because I've sat with it and learned trust and patience. It's taught me to surrender, to let go and it's invited me into flow.

I think it's only when we take the time to be still and quiet, that we can really hear it...the small quiet voice underneath all the noise.

Here are a few prompts to get you started if you haven't done it before. Take your journal and a nice pen and answer the following questions for yourself.

What do you really, really want?
What do you long to express in your life?
What do you dream of creating in your life?
What does your soul wish for at the deepest level?
What contribution would make your heart sing with joy?
How can you uncomplicate and simplify your life?
How do I make more space for what makes me happy?

MENOPAUSE – A PASSAGE TO POWER

"My sleeps gone weird" I told my Mum. "I keep waking up and I just can't get back to sleep. What's going on?". "You'll be going into the change" she said.

What? No! Not me, I do Yoga, this isn't a thing! But something was changing, my body didn't feel quite like mine anymore, my cycle was changing too. My moods were going crazy, I felt as if I was going crazy, I was all over the place. One minute I felt quite normal, the next like some kind of crazed banshee! The hot flushes started too. "I swear you're going to find me in a pile of ash on the floor one of these days" I told the kids!

It felt as if every grief I'd ever experienced came bubbling up to the surface to be dealt with too. I felt like an alien had landed and taken over my body and my mind.

Eventually, I found that while some yoga hindered, some helped. I found 'restorative and yin yoga' really helped soothe me and relaxation yoga really supported me. I realised my body needed me to slow down, to allow for this amazing process, this Rite of Passage to happen.

By that I mean, I really went into quite a dark place where all my old emotional baggage came up for me to see. All the things I'd buried arrived, especially grief, old relationships, the things I never did (like travelling and making peace with my body).

It was such a reset to look at 'Where am I in my life?' and 'Who am I becoming next?' were big questions for me. I'd been given the opportunity to heal this within me, it felt like a great remembering, a time to review my life, an invitation to heal. I hadn't realised what a beautiful process it could be, once I let go of the clutching to what had been and allowed myself to 'become'.

Once I truly surrendered to the process, I was able to move into a place of acceptance. It was truly a passage to Power.

IT'S ONLY BRICKS AND MORTAR

I remember being ready to leave, all the straws had been pulled, stamped on and broken. The last straw had been drawn! That little thing, that hadn't really seemed much but it broke the back of all the things that had gone before. It was time. Clinging onto all we had built together; it was so hard to walk away. I remember reading the poem 'If' by Rudyard Kipling and the passage 'or watch the things you gave your life to, broken and stoop and build them up with worn-out tools'. It felt mountainous!

My Dad in his wisdom said, "It's only bricks and mortar, you can't put a price on your peace of mind". There's such wisdom in that. After I walked away, the feeling of freedom was amazing and scary as hell! My life initially felt wrecked! Everyone suffered, my kids eight and sixteen years old at the time, my family, all of us were hurled into the fire.

I bought a little caravan and took it to a remote place where we went every weekend. I healed myself in nature, I got to know who I was. I'd lost so much of me; it was time to rebuild and recreate. Who am I now?

It took a couple of years to really heal, to find 'me' again. To choose you, to choose your own happiness above all else and walk away is bloody tough to navigate. To start again...it's bloody hard going. I'm not going to sit here and pretend it's easy, it's not but I can tell you without one shadow of a doubt, your happiness is worth every bit of that challenge. Choose you, it may just save your life!

MAKE SPACE FOR YOURSELF

RELAX A LITTLE MORE

My chest was tight, I couldn't breathe, my arms tingled I felt dizzy! "We'll have a Doctor out to see you soon", I heard the receptionist at the end of the phone. "It's hyperventilation due to a panic attack" the Doctor diagnosed, "I'll prescribe anti-depressants but you really need to address your stress levels". What a mess I was in!

I began looking for things to help stress, I found yoga, now an uncompromisable daily practice and my journey back to me began. Yoga soothed me, calmed my nervous system, it became my love, my life, my passion. As I tuned into the seasons and the moon cycles, I began to really feel a sense of connection and flow. Yoga had all the answers I had ever wanted to find. I found me. I became my own Guru. I got to know myself in a way that I never thought possible.

Yoga means to 'Unite – Body – Mind and Spirit', we forget the Spirit bit in our modern life and really, it's the part that just wants us to be happy, it wants us to flow, it wants the best for us. When life is overwhelming and uncertain, roll out your yoga mat, step onto it, take a breath, move your beautiful body, love your body, meet yourself just where you are and let everything else drop. Take a little time to slow down, relax, tune in to the wisdom of nature, the seasons the cycles of the moon, love yourself, accept yourself, trust yourself. Be yourself.

BE TRUE TO YOURSELF

I had a moment with Archangel Michael once. In the midst of making the hardest decision of my life, I sat in silence, asked the question, 'Should I stay or go' and the answer came as clear as day. 'I am Michael - be true to yourself'. I didn't know what it meant to be true to myself, I'd been true to everyone else but myself!

I started reading self-help books. I think Louise Hay 'The Power is Within You' was my bible for a while. I saw an advert for massage training and began a new exciting journey into yoga and holistic health. I had never dreamed it possible, I hated school and education but I had found something I loved and I spent all my time studying, I still do!

I began taking time to sit in stillness, hand on heart to listen to my inner truth and wise teacher, she has so much to say. I began asking myself questions like,

'Does this decision take me towards or away from the life I choose for me?'.
'What's the next, right move for me that would take me closer to it?'
'Am I being true to myself?'
'What would it look like if I did what I chose, what feels good?'

And sometimes it was ok for me not to have all the answers, after that experience I knew that no matter what, I could allow myself to be supported by something that was greater than me, whether I call it God, Spirit or Angel guides.

Something was holding me in love and wanted the best for me. It all worked out in the end. I'm having fun now, dreaming big and living the life I dreamed about all those years ago and I'm saying 'yes' to life every day.

You can too.

It's ok not to have
all of the answers

Lesley understands that life sometimes requires surrender, a pause and a one-step-at-a-time approach. These experiences have enriched her perspective, adding depth and value to this book.

Her voice became particularly distinct when advocating for the children she taught and their parents.

Writing her chapter was a perfectly timed opportunity. It allowed her to join a broader women's circle, an experience she cherished. In this circle, everyone shared a common objective: discovering their wise words.

With her chapter, Lesley hopes to provide nourishment and inspiration to her readers.

@nourish.nt

LESLEY MARKEY

BE KIND TO YOUR HEART, IT'S DOING AN AMAZING JOB

I had allowed myself to be broken. Surrounded by all the things... regrets, self-doubt, past mistakes, grief, fear...my world had shrunk.

My light had gone out and my heart was heavy but still, it kept beating. My beautiful heart, just doing its job in the background - protecting me, always giving and receiving love. I had to shed the weight of my heavy heart. I had to surrender to heartbreak one last time, for I believe that only when the heart truly breaks, can the light pour in.

I surrendered both my high expectations of others and of holding onto fear. I dug into those repeating patterns in friendships that were making me miserable and with a struggle, I started to let go. I started to be compassionate to myself - something I've always willingly given to others but not me.

I took a big breath and started to let it all go. With surrender came peace and peace slowly found a place in my heart. With surrender, the weight I thought was protecting my heart, lifted.

You and your heart have the amazing capacity to love. It's time to turn the love towards yourself and let your light shine.

CHANGING YOUR FOOD AT MENOPAUSE CAN FEEL SO GOOD

I changed my food routine at menopause, I felt I needed more support. I'd been studying nutrition and realised that some food 'basics' were the cornerstone to my health. Like building a house, I saw nutrition as the bricks and mortar I needed before I added the beautiful furniture!

I found that I'd been swayed by so many crazy, quick fix diets, I didn't know what were general myths or real fact at one point, there was so much information I got confused.

What helped me feel good and healthy was including protein in every meal, snacks too.

I read that we don't store it so I try to top it up at every meal. I'm also not scared of carbohydrates. I eat all the carbs, vegetables and fruits and the starchy ones too, breads and pastas, in smaller amounts.

I didn't shy away from essential, healthy fats. I eat olives, nuts and seeds, apparently seventy percent of our brains are fat based and all our cells need it. I make sure in these years I also get my vitamins in.

If you found your way to this page, maybe there's something you need to research about the food you eat. Most of us could do with knowing more and updating our knowledge base.

Once I did, I felt in control of my body. We're changing all the time. Find out what you need more of and less of, it's your beautiful body, make sure you feel good in it.

GIVE YOURSELF SOME DISTANCE, TAKE ONE STEP AT A TIME

For years, the fear of getting started kept me in the exact same spot. I'm not sure if it was the fear of failing or of not being good enough, maybe of being judged but there I was.

One day, it came to me, I was making things too complicated...too big...too un-achievable. Waiting for the perfect moment to start, I was sabotaging myself by being fearful rather than just taking one step. Too scared by the enormity of it all, I did nothing. I'd lost confidence!

I'd lost over twelve stone, I'd run half marathons, completed a total warrior, studied for post grad qualifications, all while juggling a full-time job yet my confidence had gone. I'd also been years in a job where I had no voice and couldn't be my authentic Self. I'd felt manipulated and kept small. It's hard to rebuild your confidence when you're so low but it is achievable...it just takes one step, towards what you really want.

I stepped away from that job, I didn't know what I was going to do or how to manage for money or create a new life but I did know, I couldn't stay in that job anymore. I had to give myself time and space to remember what I really wanted. If you recognise yourself in this, distance yourself from the situation that's dragging you down and remember all the things you've achieved.

You are amazing, you can do anything that you want...one step, one day at a time.

JUST STOP AND 'BE'

For years I'd filled my life with 'busy'. Rushing from work, to friends, to family, to classes, to the gym. Learning, learning, learning, doing, doing, doing, busy, busy, busy. Scared to stop. Scared to face the reality of the emptiness that was hidden within - hidden by all that rushing about!

I was scared that stopping and facing the emptiness would be my undoing. That I'd see a life without real meaning or substance, without much hope and certainly without very much joy.

I was scared to face the reality that all I'd wanted was that one special person to walk beside me, hold my hand and catch me when I fell.

I spent my life looking outwards, too scared to look within. It took me fifty-five years to realise I'd made myself busy to cover that emptiness, the feeling that I didn't fit because I wasn't meeting society norms - single and childless.

I hadn't actively sought that but I'd found myself there. Menopause, however, is a time of great reflection and nothing is really lost. The emptiness can be an amazing opportunity to discover who you really are and what you really want, so you can move into the next chapter of your life in a very different way - lit up and present with the wisdom you hold within - you just need to stop and 'be'.

NUTRITION FOR YOUR SECOND SPRING

I haven't been very good at being guided by my body in the past. Stress and grief overwhelmed me. I tried drowning out overwhelm by adding even more stress in the form of over exercising, setting up businesses and avoiding self-care. I also tried to quieten things down with foods that tasted nice but weren't doing my body any favours. I am human, not perfect; it was all a lesson.

In my second spring, I'm trying to work more with nature and what my body is telling me what I need. I'm listening to the clues about the foods she needs, switching from comfort Winter foods to the lighter/fresher foods of Spring.

I'm finding out more about nature and how women sync with the moon, even at menopause and I'm being guided by some very wise women.

In Chinese medicine, menopause is referred to as 'The Second Spring'. They recognise that if you work with nature, it can have a positive impact on your health. I love this! A new beginning, time to blossom, using nature and your body's own innate wisdom to guide the way.

I'm having a proper spring clean - out with the old - allowing space for the new. Time to blossom!

SILVER THREADS

How many times have you spoken with someone either in the real world or virtually and discovered that you have a connection? Friends in common, shared experiences, being in the same place at the same time but never meeting at any of those points? We're all connected by invisible silver threads. One of those threads has drawn you to this book and you have found yourself on this page, my page.

Those silver threads bring people and experiences into our lives just at the right time, when we have lessons to learn, growth to experience, wise wisdom to hear...a helping hand is given.

We might not recognise this at the time but these silver threads, these relationships make our lives richer. From the random conversation with a stranger or something your most cherished loved one says...silver threads bond us and make our lives complete and real. Look out for them!

STOP CHASING THE DREAM OF FRIENDSHIP

'I've left your pressie behind the bin'. A cheery message on my birthday...a gift left behind the bin. A thoughtful act of kindness or a job ticked off a list?

'I was in' I said, 'you should have knocked'. 'I didn't want to disturb you' they replied. For years, I've sent a cheery message of thanks for those presents left behind the bin and been grateful but what I really wanted was a moment of their time. It's my birthday for fucks sake, I'd think! They'd go to the effort of getting me a present but wouldn't give me a real gift of friendship, their time.

In a busy world have we got our priorities wrong? Have gifts behind bins replaced real communication and moments of friendship?

For years, I've been happy to take scraps of time and minimal effort from people I've called friends, when I've always been there for them. In the middle of the night, messaging, checking in, running around – you get the idea.

But there's been a shift. I've stopped. I've shed so many tears, thinking that the friendship was more than it ever was. My message to you, is stop! Stop chasing the dream of friendship and look at the reality of the true friends around you. Let go, with love, those who are only in your life for their own means.

WHAT I WISH I HAD KNOWN BEFORE MENOPAUSE

I didn't really think about it until it happened. I was so lucky, the first time I went through it, it was rather a non-event. Apparently around 20% of us will sail through menopause - no symptoms - no big earth-shattering life changing event. Just 'Oh, I've not had a period for over a year, that must be me done then!'

But my body had other ideas. It had kept the score of years of stress at work, when I'd pushed it to the max with exercise and yo-yo dieting and it was going to have the final word!

BOOM burnout and work-related anxiety that had me off work for nine months with the unions involved, pushed me back into perimenopause but this time with rapid weight gain, sleeplessness, hot sweats and brain fog!

It was a nightmare. If you're setting out on your menopause journey, the kindest thing you can do for your body is to reduce your stress, allowing your adrenal glands the capacity of producing oestrogen and progesterone, supporting the reduction of menopausal symptoms.

Not dealing with stress keeps your body primed for attack, drives blood pressure up and slows down other systems like digestion and metabolism, leaving you open to increased risk of heart attack, stroke as well as weight gain and digestive problems. Dealing with stress will ease your transition through menopause - setting you up for a healthier midlife.

Mairi has come to know, love and accept herself for the unique individual she is. Her voice has got stronger, allowing her to be heard as a friend, daughter, partner and business owner.

"When my voice comes from a place of aligned love" she says, "it's most definitely heard!"

She wrote her chapter as part of her personal evolution and to develop and strengthen her voice even further.

@mairitaylor_menopause_rockstar

MAIRI TAYLOR

HONOUR THE GRIEF

Today I cried in the Post Office. I popped in and saw posters everywhere informing us that the Post Master had unexpectedly died. His wife was working away behind the counter serving customers and getting people's prescriptions and that simply broke the flood gates open! As I started to cry, the lady behind the counter looked at me very perplexed. I took a deep breath, finished my transaction and burst into tears, walking away, letting all my pent-up grief pour out.

When my sister died, I went back to work the next day. What else was I going to do other than sit and look at the flowers my colleagues had sent me? My mum was thousands of miles away, where my sister had died and they'd had the chance to have the kinds of conversations that tidied up any messiness in their relationship.

Mum and I had never really spoken about the impact of Sarah's death. We chose not to. Our grief was hidden and private, rather than being a shared gift to each other.

Slowly, our relationship eroded and we spoke even less. Now I can't speak to her again or hear her answers to the many questions I have. So I sit with, not just the grief of the loss of my sister, of my father and my mother (her Alzheimer's is too far gone now) but the conversations and milestones we'll never celebrate together.

Oh, to have one last conversation, to ask that one question, to honour the grief and sink into it exploring and honouring it together.

If you too find yourself in this space all I can say is ask for help. You don't have to walk this path alone. Please know that in time, you can have those difficult conversations around grief. 'Keeping calm and carrying on', pushing and stuffing your emotions down, self-soothing with your 'drug' of choice serves no-one, especially not you.

Find that safe space where you can be seen, heard and HELD without anyone trying to fix or rationalise your emotions or your grief, because that's what they are...yours and no-one is allowed to diminish you.

Allowing yourself to live a full and vibrant life may be the bets way to honour the light and life of those no longer dancing with you.

SAYING NO IS THE BEST SELF CARE ADVICE

I dare you to say 'No', next time you're asked to do something that doesn't resonate deeply with you. As a reforming people pleaser, brought up in a society which applauded 'good girls', 'sugar and spice and all things nice', it's been very hard for me to learn the subtle art of simply saying no.

> 'No thank you, that's not for me'.
> 'No thank you, I'm not available',
> 'No thank you, I don't have time'.

You may have spent most of your life saying yes to things you didn't really want to do, buying things you didn't want, over indulging and over giving because nobody taught you to honour your space, thoughts and needs. We live in a society that's happiest when women show up as compliant and subservient, serving the coffee, putting everyone's needs before ours. It's no wonder there's a backlash against the silver haired queen's saying no, standing in their power, reclaiming their space!

AND, it's not just the silver haired queens, young women are challenging societal norms and showing us the way!

By saying NO to additional requests on your time, you're saying YES to you! Try it! Blame your menopause I don't care, simply start saying YES to you and teach others that your needs are as deserving as theirs and you may just find out who you are.

SURRENDER

It was December 2020, I was laying face down on the floor and a group of women were dancing all around me, the only word I kept hearing was 'Surrender'. All I knew, was that that word resonated with every cell in my body!

It was time. Time to stop running at life, time to stop the busyness, yes even during global down time I could stay busy but what I really needed, was to surrender to me, my life and the process of my Menopause transition. It was time to stop controlling and simply allow life to unfurl.

I'm a woman of the eighties...shoulder pads, big hair and 'show me the money' was all in. The purpose of life back then, was to be 'faster', 'more' and flatline what it meant to be a woman, with a cycle of shifting energies.

Most of us went along for the ride. We were told we could have everything, when actually, that was so far from the truth. Many of us are only now unpicking those messages as we hit the door of Menopause like a brick, wondering why we're feeling let down by our bodies and minds.

Our bodies have not let us down, we were misinformed, uneducated and led astray by those who didn't actually understand what it meant to be a woman. It's time to surrender now and give back to her. I'm doing exactly that.

Take it easy, step back, surrender and let it all be easy, I think it really is.

THE BUTTERFLY EFFECT

For a caterpillar to transform into a butterfly, they have to allow themselves to turn in to the most glorious goop. Imaginal cells create the butterfly the caterpillar was always destined to be. If anyone tries to hurry that process or help the butterfly emerge, their lives are shortened and they don't get to live their full glorious next phase of life.

What if your menopause transition is your glorious gloopy phase? A full breakdown of the woman you are, in order to become the woman you're meant to be, in the next chapter of your life.

It's a true 'unbecoming'. We have to allow the gloopy mess, where everything we thought we were disintegrates, in order to create the glorious new versions of ourselves.

We can't rush it, force it or deny it. Doing so, would impact the quality and vibrancy of the next phase, it would be like dishonouring the woman you were and the woman you are yet to know.

What if we could all enter this phase of life allowing the breakdowns, the reimagining and the gloopy, sticky mess? What if we saw, heard and felt it for what it was? What if we knew that allowing this mess would mean we emerged as newly formed women who would open our wings and fly! Menopause creates a new sense of freedom, it'll take you to the next chapter!

If you've opened this page here, I invite you to go find your army of caterpillars, those fellow beings who will honour and acknowledge your gloopy mess with love...those beings who know that 'this too will pass', whilst gifting you the time and space to just 'be in the gloop'. You can emerge in your own time and in your own way, into a kaleidoscope of butterflies, flying free together.

TRACK YOUR CYCLE WITH THE MOON

As I've sunk deeper into my own post-menopause journey, my rage against the patriarchal system has grown, I've learned that many doctors have had no training whatsoever in our menopause. The deeper my learning has gone, the more I'm outraged by how women's health is treated. I feel we've been belittled by the whole system.

But rather than raging against it, I gathered that rage within myself and I got educated. I reconnected with my body and my cycle and I honour the messages she gives me every minute of every day!

I started with the moon. She's our guiding light in terms of tuning into our energy, mood, sleep and sociability. Look up at the next New or Full Moon and track your body, your cycle and your moods and energy. You'll notice patterns in your behaviour that run in tandem with her cycle.

This means that by getting quiet and listening day-by-day to your body's whispers, moon cycle by moon cycle, you will start to reconnect with the woman you are becoming and find your way home, by the light of the moon.

UNPACK THE BOXES

I genuinely thought I would green juice and weightlift my way through menopause! Eat well, take the supplements, move my body...but a decade ago, I read a quote from Dr Christiane Northrup and it resonated so deeply with me...

Menopause is a time when we may come up against the unfinished business that we have accumulated over the first half of our life. We may find ourselves grieving for losses never fully grieved. It is as if we have gone down to the basement and found boxes and boxes of things to be sorted and weeded out"

Seven years later, I truly understood what that meant as I came to fully appreciate the impact of years of submerged feelings, all wanting to be seen, heard and felt.

My menopause symptoms weren't just a result of physical changes but of trauma and chronic stress too. My heart heard the call all those years ago and then on the cusp of my menopause, I started to slowly unpack the boxes, weeding through the emotions to remove what was not mine or no longer of service.

It was a gift to my body, to my heart and soul. I was finding the peace they needed to bring my body back to a place of balance. Unpacking the boxes is not to be rushed. You may have to wait patiently, as you sit in the void, trusting the process. It will take as long as it takes. Maybe you'll journal, maybe you'll talk it out, maybe you'll go outside and walk in nature.

Maybe you'll dance, meditate or whatever the FLIP you need to do to unpack those boxes. Maybe you'll do all of these things over and over again until you know you've totally unpacked what needs unpacking. This is a time of patience. You'll find your way to the other side and come back home to you.

WE DON'T NEED MORE PUMPS, WE NEED LESS STRESS

Recently, I've been talking to women about their hormone replacement therapy journeys. I've been on my own three-month journey with body identical hormone replacement therapy and I'm hearing women saying they feel the need to take more pumps of oestrogen to manage their ongoing or increasing menopause symptoms.

I'm also hearing worry as they know they're already prescribed maximum dose. I asked one lady, 'What changed this month?', she explained her work load had increased dramatically, plus a few extra add-ons involving looking after everyone else and then she apologised for 'making a fuss'! I don't think we need extra pumps, I think we need less stress!

I believe many of us are carrying a load that's overwhelming, leading to enhanced symptoms of menopause. If you found your way to this page, this is your permission to put your load down, stop mothering everyone else and start mothering yourself. Show unconditional love for you to get the best OF you, you deserve to have your needs met too!

YOUR HISTORY IS NOT YOUR DESTINY

I'm not sure if it was a conscious decision to make the choices I did but I do remember the moment I realised that I was the healthiest member of my family! I questioned why – was I here to stop the cycle? I've been surrounded by family illness, yet approaching mid-life, I'm fit and well. The daughter/granddaughter of Alzheimer's, my sister died of cancer at twenty-eight, my dad died in his fifties to alcohol, my grandparents never reached seventy and yet I'm healthy.

And while I questioned that, I did notice that I have never felt fearful of disease, it has simply motivated me to look after myself more. I've made lifestyle choices to minimise the 'switching on' of genes and I deeply trust my body to look after me, as I look after her, always have, always will. Epigenetics is the study of how our behaviours and environment causes changes in the way our genes work. When I compare my lifestyle to my mother's, I can see I'm intentionally steering the course of my destiny.

Your health history is not your destiny. Reducing your toxic load through your food, your products and your thoughts can all positively impact your inner environment. It's never too late to change your destiny.

Jan wrote her chapter with the intention of collaborating with other women. She believes in the power of collective action, proclaiming, "When we act together, a woman's voice becomes a revolution!"

Much like you, Jan has navigated the challenge of finding and asserting her voice. She has been an advocate for numerous individuals, particularly in the realm of pregnancy and childbirth. She's fearlessly championed the rights of young people to be acknowledged in their unique diversity and she's campaigned for their equality within the community and educational system.

Jan's chapter comes directly from her heart. Her aspiration is for her words to guide you towards your happiness, empowering you to stay true to yourself.

JAN CALVERT

USE YOUR VOICE

I always wanted to feel the wind in my hair. I would ride my bike home from school down the big hill as fast as I dared. I loved it most when it was about to rain, a proper throw down, the air heavy with that rush of an impending storm, to ride home, beating the clouds before they broke.

As a teenager I marched for Women's rights and campaigned for Amnesty. I wanted to stick two fingers up to those who annoyed me, burn bridges and stand up for my rights. I'd challenge authority, play Bob Marley, Janis Joplin and dream with John Lennon. A freedom fighter, I've always had a strong feeling that being 'me' necessitates that I AM FREE.

When I tried to 'fit in' and quieten my voice, it would erupt, speak out, react against injustice. If I tried to keep my voice down, it ended up revolting...like voltage...hot words loading and ready to fire.

So...I use my voice better now, more often, to avoid explosion, I use my passion and courage. When we all find our voices and say what we need to, we stand together, we defend our earth.

A woman's voice has a right to be heard, we are a revolution!

FIND THE THINGS YOUR MUM TAUGHT YOU, IN THE BEST OF HER TIMES AND THE WORST

In my experience, mothers and daughters can be both best friends and spiky judges. I feel we expect so much of our mothers, that when they let us down, it can provoke more anger and pain than any other relationship let down.

My relationship with my mother, was at times, fraught with expectation and disappointment. When I stopped such unfair expectations of her, we became good friends.

I gained my sense of independence from her. She took me to Africa when I was just ten weeks old, back then that was a big deal!

As an adult, I've followed that same independence, I've hitch-hiked through Europe, stayed in a beautiful commune in Amsterdam and travelled through Oman. It's from her that I gained my love of nature and thirst for knowledge, for me, for herbs and homeopathy, healing energy and reiki.

I learned the importance of good friends, a decent book and a sunny step. She told me to 'choose my battles', do what I wanted, not to worry and that it'd all be ok!

Her life had its ups and downs but she seemed to forget the bad stuff and simply remember the good. I learned to see the beauty in life from her, I learned to both live it up and also to stand still, for just another moment, beneath a blossom tree.

Mum taught me the names of flowers and trees. She believed in angels and had a depth of kindness that is so rare. Impulsive and reckless, she left large scatterings of memories that still make me laugh and cry, I never really appreciated my mum until she died.

Whatever your relationship with your mum, choose to remember the beautiful things she taught you – whether it be through her great example or her worst behaviour – she will have passed wisdom to you, it's time to find it.

Your mind is not you, it's yours to look after

As I walk through the silver birch and oak woodland, the smell of wild garlic and the nod of new bluebells take me to a stiller world. The sunlight dapples through the leaves and I feel peace.

The traffic of my mind slows down and a wider expanse of peacefulness opens up. To detach and observe, is a lifelong discipline and practice for me. To stand back and let thoughts go, releasing me from the chaotic ramblings and interior chatter, the negative self-talk and incessant social concerns.

The mind is intricate and interesting but the voice within our heads is not always our friend. I say aloud, 'Stop that now' to cease the pest: there's no need to berate oneself, judge or complain, just let it go and allow it to drift on by.

When the mind is quiet, the soul can radiate its golden light, topping up from Source, filling with love once more. The mind needs a spring clean sometimes, an assessment of its content from time to time or it can take over.

It's our responsibility to prune it back, weed out the rubbish and deter the parasitic pests. It is ours to choose, what to keep and what we can let go of. Your mind is not you – it's yours to look after.

HANG IN THERE

'Ten thousand sorrows, and ten thousand joys' Chuang Tzu

I have three children. And I have three more who didn't live full-term to birth. My womb has brought me both the greatest of joys and the deepest of sadness.

The midwife pulled cold gel across the stillness of my belly and searched the screen. There was no heartbeat. Crying, I left the hospital and carried the heavy news home. I had yet to give birth to my baby and I knew the pain that came a few days later, meant it was time for me and my body to let her go.

A year on from that and we found ourselves carrying a tiny, white coffin into the Chapel of Rest thanking our next child for being with us, if only for such a very short time. The third was sooner and less physically traumatic but part of me hid, deep within my grief, surfacing only to care for my children, to do the daily tasks, go to work and to brave the playground.

Around me, the children searched for treasure, climbed trees and played with magic sticks. We learnt to fly, jumping with batman wings from rocks and making flowery potions. The light seeped in: smiles warmed me, strong women held me and I pushed away the shadows. In time, my eldest daughter had a baby! I was with her when my grandson was born: what happiness and joy. My heart was filled.

In a woman's life, in your life, there will be 10,000 tears of sorrow. Hang in there please. Time does heal and balance is restored, for we all do also have our 10,000 tears of joy.

BE A FREE SPIRIT BUT KEEP YOUR FEET FIRMLY ON THE FLOOR

Three days after my twenty-third birthday, I became a Mum and have brought up my daughter alone. My love for my kids has been my inspiration, they mean everything to me. I'm a free spirit but had to keep my feet firmly on the floor. In school, I liked ska and two tone but was a hippy at heart. In my dreams, I wore flowers in my hair and 'Imagine' was my manifesto.

When I did my maths O'Level I wrote 'Don't divide: Share', at the bottom of the paper and gained a B. I'm forever thankful for my grounded education and that I've been able to work and support my family. I'm glad the times-table was drilled into me as I've navigated the family finances keeping our heads just about above water. I trained to be a teacher and worked full-time, it was exhausting and I was buzzing, I felt so proud and inspired by my love for my daughter.

Every day I'd wake filled with determination and say my mantra: 'You're getting there Jan, you're getting there!'.

I think of the strong women who came before me, their strong voices, determination to survive, their independent and fulfilling lives...my great, great auntie was a suffragette, one grandma was a teacher, the other a midwife.

It's wonderful to be a free spirit but I've also learnt the practicalities to make it work, keeping my feet firmly grounded on the floor!

DO JUST WHAT YOU WANT!

My Grandad died when I was just five and my Grandma lived in grief. She kept it quietly and firmly inside of her. Her first daughter also died before her, of Polio and everyone loved a little less after that.

My cousins and I were born into this very well-established family of 'silent grief' and instinctively, we knew not to disturb it. We tiptoed around under the stern eyes of
our heart-hardened parents. But the last time I saw my Grandma, she said something to me I never expected to hear.

"Do what YOU want Jan", she said, "just smile sweetly and get on with it". I'd never seen that mischievous side of her before. I was a mother and hadn't married and Grandma not only seemed to approve of me but she seemed delighted.

I remember her clapping and laughing as my daughter ran around her garden, jumping on the paving stones under the washing line. I wish I could have played with her like that when I was a child, I could have shone rays of light through her fragmented grief - if only I hadn't 'done as I was told'. It's better to enjoy life and do just what you want!

LOVE YOURSELF A LITTLE MORE

There are some things I regret...

- I regret passing time with people who saw me but didn't know me.
- I regret that I didn't follow my heart and instead did what worked best for others.
- I regret my delusions and romantic notions; the naiveties of a shy and tender heart...wiser eyes would have served me better and perhaps, yes, a more cynical heart.

It's true...I have allowed another to be untruthful with me, to disrespect and to use me. I haven't spoken up.

I've crumpled like discarded litter in the corner of the yard. I lost belief in myself. I let my strength be sapped. My lonely intuition cried out to me unheard.

But when I remember those times, I also remember that we must rise up! I have a word with myself: 'Let it go! Don't berate yourself. It is done. Learn the lesson and move on.'

We're here to live and to love, these are the times we must love ourselves just a little more.

TAKE A ROAD TRIP!

The Scottish Highlands are stunningly beautiful. I have an old MX5 and when the roof is down and the sky is blue, it feels like I'm in heaven!

My youngest two were both off to university and I'd just celebrated my fifty-fifth birthday. This was to be a time of transition. Part of me felt thrilled and liberated - for the first time in my adult life it seemed, I could do exactly as I pleased. Part of me is proud, I've worked towards this point, as all parents do, to see my children safely through the passage of their childhood into independence and adulthood. Each of them an individual, full of their own insights and wisdom. They make me laugh out loud. They are my favourite people.

And now, I need to prepare for my own future, a time without the responsibilities and daily workload of a family at home. It's unsettling. My time is less defined. I must now unwrap the layers of the years and see what pieces of me remain relevant. Who am I now as I pass through the menopause and into a time of my own?

I chose my CDs, took the dog and set off on a thousand miles of alone time. My destination: the ancient and mystical island of Orkney. Scary, liberating and fabulously fun! Life is a journey. Take a road trip!

Stepping into her role as the crone, Stevie has used her voice her whole life to stand up for herself and for others. She has fiercely protected her daughters, fought for the home birth she wanted all those years ago and more recently, advocated for the care her husband needed.

As a special needs teacher, she speaks up on behalf of her students too, ensuring they are seen and respected.

Her female inspirations have been her mum, Barbara and a very special teacher, Daisy Oates. Now, writing for this book of women over fifty, she says, "The crone voice needs to be heard." We are very pleased she joined this powerful book of wise women!

@sjwangel

STEVIE FOSTER

CREATE RITUAL

We all have daily habits: the morning cup of coffee, our route to work, our daily three pm pick me up! Habits become life enhancing rituals when we do them with more intention though.

My morning hot water and lemon became a joyful ten-minute ritual when I starting making it in my favourite tea pot, covered with my glorious tea cosy that looks like grass and has crocheted bees and sunflowers on it!

I pour my lemony water into my favourite mug and I sip slowly and imagine all the good things it's doing in my body.

I love creating and working with ritual. In my yoga room I've created a number of little altars that help me set my intentions and work with ritual in a focused way. I have an altar that changes with the seasons and cycles of the year. On there, I place objects I've found on my walks and I honour the elements of earth, fire, air and water.

I have an altar that honours my yoga journey and the special gifts I've been given. A heart shaped tray is dedicated to love. On there are all sorts of heart shaped objects. Every ritual I do is focused on love.

I'm working with the goddess Kali at the moment and I have an altar honouring her. A central tray table at the perfect height, to sit at during meditation. This has the 'tools of the trade' on it...candles, incense, a tiny bell, a beautiful ceramic rattle, my cacao cup, crystals and other special objects that I use daily.

Ritual brings me joy, it's as simple as that.

ALLOW YOURSELF TO BE ENCHANTED BY NATURE

Over the years I have, at times, felt completely disconnected from the natural world. I've been caught up in mind numbing domestic drudgery or terrible anxiety depending on where my children were at!

I remember going out for a walk one day and not being able to identify the season we were in. Happily, now I am completely enchanted by the nature around me.

Walking to work used to be a route march, now I take my time and stop to find the woodpecker I can hear in the trees or look at the buds forming or stare in fascination at a new kind of fungi I have never seen before. You will find me talking to squirrels, rabbits, birds and trees. I pick things up from the ground and put them in my pocket and I'm delighted when I find these little treasures again weeks later.

People ask me if I get bored walking the same way all the time and visiting the same park on my early morning walks but I find it so soothing to my soul to be intimately connected with the world around me. I know every bush and tree.

I look forward to the natural order of snow drops, then crocuses, then daffodils, then wild garlic, then bluebells. I'm fascinated by the ebb and flow of the beck through the seasons.

Wind, rain and snow can all cause havoc but I love to check in with my favourite places after an extreme weather event and see how things have changed. I have learnt to actively let go of the chatter in my mind and fully immerse myself in the here and now. I savour the sights, smells, touch and occasionally the taste of my environment. I have come home.

PRACTICE SELF-MASSAGE

I flirted with self-massage for years and about five years ago committed to a daily practice. I don't mean rubbing a bit of cream into my body after a shower, I consider self-massage a part of my daily spiritual practice, alongside drinking ceremonial cacao, moving my body, meditating, receiving and savouring.

I make up essential oil blends to suit my body, the time of year and my general mood. I slowly massage the oil into every part of my body. I use energy medicine techniques, I work with the energy channels of the body to soothe or energise depending on my need.

This daily practice has done more to help me love my body than any other practice. Listening to what my body needs and responding to it with loving and gentle touch has allowed me to let go of ingrained hatred towards my shape and how I felt it had let me down over the years.

I don't just accept my body now. I haven't just come to terms with the fact that I will never have a flat stomach. I love my body and I honour it for everything it does for me. I am actively embracing the ageing process and am fascinated by the changes in my body. I can't wait to see what will happen next.

It has taken me years to feel this way about my body but the very simple practice of self-massage has been a beautiful journey. I highly recommend it.

CARVE SOME TIME OUT FOR YOURSELF EVERY DAY

I was twenty-one and working in a hotel in Maine, my job was stressful, the guests we served in the restaurant every evening were extremely demanding, I'd feel so nervous, every single day before I went to work.

As a young employee, I lived in and while my colleagues would stay by the pool until the last possible moment before their shift, I couldn't...I started doing yoga before I went to work every day. I would shower and then do twenty minutes or so of yoga and breathing. I found that it made a huge difference to my anxiety.

Over the years, I've kept this up, committing to a practice of yoga and meditation every morning. I think this saved my life, my sanity and my marriage. It certainly became the solid foundation on which I have built my rich and beautiful daily spiritual practice.

Essentially, I've made sure I've had time for myself. When the children were little, I'd spend time studying, I trained to be a homeopath, I managed one blissful weekend a month to focus on a subject I found fascinating and completely life enhancing! Later, I trained to be a yoga teacher to make the most of my precious early morning time too. Carve out time for yourself every single day, it's worth every second, if you're waiting for a permission slip, consider this it!

LOOK AT THE MOON!

I love the moon. If you look at my social media pages, you won't find very much but you will find lots of terrible photographs I've taken of the moon with the caption 'Look at the moon!'.

I've spent the last year studying the moon, the astronomy and astrology, how ancient people related to the moon in their rituals and ceremonies. I've learned how it relates to the seasons and cycles and its relationship to the goddesses.

All of this is fascinating but really I just love looking at the moon! I get a thrill of excitement when I see the full moon rise. I'm completely enthralled when I'm on my early morning walks and the sun and the moon are in the sky at the same time. The sheer magnificence of this event is amazing to me.

My husband indulges my weirdness gracefully but even he gets my fascination with the moon. On our first big trip in our camper van, we spent two delightful evenings in a pub garden watching a super full moon rise. We were both mesmerised by this stunning sight.

Last night I was sitting in my front room and hadn't yet closed the curtains, suddenly the clouds parted and there was the bright sliver of the new moon and Venus shining brightly underneath. Stunning! Just go and look at the moon!

MOVE YOUR BODY

I love nothing more than putting on a piece of music and letting my body move me. So often we think we move the body but I let it move me instead. I just let it happen, no pushing, no expectations. Just listening deeply to needs of my body and letting it flow. This sort of movement is deeply nourishing to the body, mind and spirit.

I actually dislike exercise for the sake of exercise but I have always loved movement...ballet classes, ice skating when I started school, I'm from Nottingham, in the UK, so everyone wanted to be Torvill and Dean!

For many years I trained as an ice dancer, I never really considered it exercise, I loved pushing my body to do all sorts of amazing things like spins and jumps, putting together sequences to music.

Yoga has been my main stay over the years but I've experimented with lots of different styles of dance, Tai Chi, Qigong, Pilates and Spirit dance. Having an embodied movement practice is really important to me; I feel I do what my body is asking for, rather than moving 'correctly' or in the prescribed way.

Embodied movement is a truly sensory experience, flowing and fun.

SENSES ARE A MAGIC PORTAL TO FULFILMENT

As a yoga teacher I studied yoga philosophy, translated and interpreted by western men. If these philosophers are to be believed, then the senses are bad things that lead us into temptation. They say it's vital that we move away from the temptations of the body and only this will allow us to achieve enlightenment. I spent years in meditation, trying to master my mind and withdraw my senses. A few years ago, I started to question this approach.

I am a human being. I have chosen to be a human being for a reason. Surely, I need to be working with my body, not against it. What if I actually tried to cultivate my senses? I tried it with my morning cuppa. I held the cup in my hands and received the scent of the tea. I imagined that every cell in my body had a smell receptor and could savour the scent of my tea with every cell.

Try it...feel the warmth of the cup in your hands. Really savour that sensation on your skin, sip your tea and savour the flavour in your mouth, on your tongue, in your throat. Imagine, as I did, that every cell in your body can taste the liquid and savour every molecule. Let your eyes rest on something in the room and savour the light, the shapes, the colours.

Take it all in without reaching or grasping, just receive every sensation. In this way I have found I enter the moment. I am completely fulfilled by every small and simple detail. This practice has helped me to feel so much more satisfied with my everyday life. I'm no longer grasping for the next thing to make me happy, I'm happy with what I find.

WALK TOWARDS THE RISING SUN

According to Ayurveda, walking towards the rising sun every morning is a cure for depression. Walking for me has been a source of solace for many years. I have a very emotionally demanding job and when my children were teenagers, my home life was pretty demanding too.

Walking to work and back gave me the space I needed between home and work/work and home, to let go of what had been during the day and prepare for what was to come. A few years back, I had an overwhelming desire not only to walk every day but to walk towards the rising sun. I got up just before dawn and set out towards the sun every day.

Of course, as the year progressed, I got up earlier and earlier but this never became a chore. I absolutely loved the quiet, calm early morning. There's something very special about greeting the sun every morning along with all of nature.

I felt so much more connected to nature and the seasons and cycles of the earth. I felt like I had a place there and that I was anchored, even when all around me seemed to be falling apart.

I was delighted to see all sorts of animals which I wouldn't usually see at busier times of the day like deer, herons, king fishers and my all-time favourite sighting – otters! I can truly say that walking towards the rising sun has changed my life.

As a journalist, Suzy has expressed herself through writing. However, she candidly admits, "learning to stand up for myself has been the longest journey."

Immersed in the collective energy of wise women while sharing her wisdom has been a 'glorious' experience for her.

She aspires that her words, her encouragement and her stories instill hope within you — a hope that you, too, can firmly stand up for yourself like she does now!

@iamsuzywalker

SUZY WALKER

JUST BE RIGHT HERE, RIGHT NOW

When I was sixteen, I sat in a ward that smelt of disinfectant and cabbage, with squeaky trolleys rolling by every ten seconds that gibbered the beside of my dad who was dying of stomach cancer. He was helping me revise for my O levels and he was testing me on chemistry equations. "How many did I get right?", "2 out of 37!". "I'm going to fail," I wailed to him, as only a self-obsessed teen could do, sitting at the bedside of her dying father.

"It doesn't matter, baby. None of it matters," he would say, trying to hold my hand but failing because his energy ran out. He died not long after that conversation. Three years later, my mum died too. It was a bit of a shock to the system to lose my parents when I was a teenager. 'To lose one parent, Mr Worthing, may be regarded as a misfortune; to lose both looks like carelessness,' wrote one famous writer.

I decided not to be careless with my life. I made big leaps, I trained as a journalist and then as a coach, learning to ask big questions like – 'What makes my heart leap?' 'What does matter?' and 'What do I care about?'. What I discovered, is that life isn't about gaining enough knowledge to pass a test so you can get to some future destination that will (hopefully) bring you happiness but it's about learning how to love and accept yourself and others. It's about how to find ways to be 'right here, right now' in the present...because ultimately that's all we ever have. My dad was right. None of the other stuff does matter.

FOCUS ON WHAT MAKES YOUR HEART LEAP, NOT WHO

'I'm in love,' my friends say. 'My commiserations,' I reply. Experts say that falling in love is a rush of chemicals scarily similar to those on our best ever 'dance-on-the bar-Tequila-shot' nights out! You're flying, invincible, indestructible but don't be fooled. It's a trick of nature to keep us mating and procreating. It doesn't last. Your obsession with their curly eyelashes, their every word and their breath on your neck, fades.

Those feelings last up to two years, a glorious and agonising ride, the truth is, it's not about them, it's about you. All that talk about 'finding your other half' and 'you complete me' is a load of old bollocks!

You have to be your own other half, you have to complete you! It's wonderful to have a companion, a warm body in your bed but the truth is, Orson Welles was right. 'We're born alone, we die alone.' Harsh, but liberating.

Once you realise that, you can stop looking to others to make you feel better and look to yourself instead. Stop giving all your power away to someone else and fill your own holes...so-to-speak! I'm not saying you shouldn't look for a partner but rather than been guided by the chemical rush of seeing their curves, find out what makes you tick first. What lights you up? What makes your heart leap?

Notice what you find yourself doing when no-one else is watching, what you're interested in and what draws your attention. Who you admire and why? What you love and what you do effortlessly are your life values! Identify those and then seek out others who share them. Then once the hangover of lust kicks in, you'll have someone to enjoy the fry-up with the next morning!

YOU CAN DO THIS!

"I can do this" I say out loud. I stand alone in my wheelhouse, (that's the back bit of the canal boat I'd just moved onto.) Supporting my sixteen-year-old son to go to Sixth Form in London, we couldn't afford the extortionate rents or train fares to London, so I'd been creative and moved us onto a forty-five-foot canal boat.

I'd never sailed before. "You don't sail a canal boat, you motor it", said a mansplainer in the 'Canal Boating for beginners' online group. The previous owner had kindly sellotaped lots of drawings to the cupboards of what to pull and push, I'd been studying YouTube videos on how to 'motor' a canal boat for weeks. But the moment was now here. My stomach clenched...'You are a strong, capable, intelligent woman, you can do this!'.

In situations like this, it's not your adult self who needs reassuring, it's your inner waif, the one who wails and gets hysterical when faced with new challenges. I have the theory that we all need re-parenting – or maybe it's just me?

Everyone needs encouragement, some are lucky to learn that from parents or teachers, some were bought up with 'the little engine who could' as bedtime reading. And some of us are late to that party!

Adulthood provides us with the opportunities to give ourselves the encouragement we didn't get as children. Every scary challenge is an opportunity to coax, reassure and motivate your inner waif. Life is hard enough without listening to our inner critic...choose another voice, 'I am loved and supported', 'I am lucky', 'I can motor this canal boat into Central London when I've never done it before!' and I did!

YOU ARE STRONG AND CAPABLE

LISTEN TO YOUR EMOTIONS

I was so hungover I vomited into my woolly hat in the back of the taxi in front of my boss. I was in my twenties and had been drinking far too much on a regular basis. My boss was a wise old bird. She didn't sack me but gave me her therapist's number.

Her therapist told me I must make my emotions my friend. "They're trying to tell you something" she said. She was right. If you try to numb your emotions, they just get louder and louder until you do eventually hear them. The alcohol (or the binge-eating or the working too hard or whatever may be your drug of choice) can only soothe you for so long. It can only help you numb things until they creak and bend, eventually cascading, shattering into a million pieces, leaving your shell broken on the floor.

"But know it's only the shell", said the therapist. Beneath that protective layer is you. Sometimes the shell gets broken prematurely, your wings aren't fully formed, so you're a little fragile and weak. But if the wind is in the right direction and you have some kind people to help, then you slowly build your muscles and get stronger and you'll learn how to fly.

I learned that it's wise to seek out kind people to help you and never to mistake the shell for your life...then learning to fly is much easier.

SCAMBUST YOUR OWN SCAMS

Beware your 'scams'. Our scams are essentially the systems we created to keep ourselves safe as children. My favourite scam was 'poor, brave me'. I was the world's favourite martyr. I did everything for everyone else. I was a giving friend, a dutiful daughter and wife who supported her husband financially and emotionally. And how was I? 'Fine, if a little resentful...'. I'd set this scam up in childhood and at some point, I'd made the decision that love was conditional and I would have to do A, B and C to be loved.

The way I chose to get the love I wanted, was by being a giver and a martyr. I'd clean the house for my parents, be the good one who didn't stay out late, I was the sweet, 'good girl' of the family. As an adult, I was twitchy with resentment, screening calls because my friends were always ringing me to dump their problems but never asked about mine, plus I resented supporting my husband to live his dreams when I was left at home in Cinderella mode. It was time for what I call 'scambusting'. It's very liberating. Firstly, I had to identify the scam...'What was I doing that no longer served me?'.

Once I found the scam, I had to look at the payoffs and costs of it on my health, temper, resilience and energy. For me, I had to believe I was loveable for just being me.

Slowly, I began to look for concrete evidence that that was true and slowly things began to change. Yes, I lost a few friends (and a husband) but suddenly I got better jobs, found new friends and I felt very loved.

YOU ARE ABSOLUTELY GOOD ENOUGH!

Twenty-five years ago, I woke up. I woke up thirty miles from home at the end of the tube line, having slept through my stop and thought 'I can't do this anymore.' I was working sixteen hours a day, six days a week, grind, grind, non-stop. I was tired. All the time.

My whole day was spent fighting a bone-crushing fatigue that seemed to eat me up from the inside out until all I could do was cushion myself on the sofa every night lest the slightest knock shattered me into tiny, brittle pieces.

I hired a coach. She asked me what life I wanted to create for myself and then asked the question that changed my life. "What would you have to believe about yourself for this dream to come true?". I blustered, I sneered, I sneered a bit more but, in the end, I wept. I realised that to create a life I loved, I was going to have change me. It was an inside job. I had to build my confidence, my belief in myself and find ways to champion myself versus always pulling myself down.

If you don't believe you're good enough, if you listen to the voice of fear, what happens is, you can't say 'no'. You put up with stuff you shouldn't and you work day and night to prove you're worthy of a place in the world.

When I stopped looking to the outside world to validate me and championed myself instead, life became a lot more enjoyable. I found fun and peace and (fortunately) I no longer fall asleep on the tube!

What do you want instead?

Krysia and Sarah have been wise, gracious and gentle influences on Tamsyn in her journey to find her purpose and voice.

She says she was always strongly in her masculine energy, demanding people hear her but now recognises that her "clearest voice is actually much quieter and more gentle". She has softened into her feminine strength, allowing her authentic voice to emerge.

She notes, "It is noticeable how much more often I am deeply heard and witnessed now".

She wrote her chapter for many reasons...one of which was to practice writing 'as herself' in a safe environment. She hopes you will find support, love, understanding and compassion in her words.

@tamsyn.synergease

TAMSYN STANTON

STAY INTERESTED AND ADVENTUROUS

I am truly grateful to all the glorious women who showed me what it might look like to age gracefully, in good health, with my mental acuity intact. Those women have given me the impetus to eat well, exercise regularly, keep my brain active by constantly learning new things and they've inspired me to explore whatever ignites my interest. They dress in bright colours, dye their hair vivid shades, learn how to dance Salsa, climb mountains and run marathons.

It was a massive milestone when I passed fifty. Vibrant and excited by life, I realised I was still anticipating new adventures and changes of direction. I've had ups and downs, times when I've wondered what the point of it all was. I have no parents and no children, no partner, it's just me and my little dog. But then I find a new hobby, make new friends and get enthused all over again.

A few years ago, while working as ambulance crew, I trained to be a hypnotherapist and qualified as a Certified Zentangle Teacher, I also passed more Standup Paddleboard instructor courses.

I qualified as an Aura Mediator to do Aura Transformations for others and as the course was in Scotland (several hundred miles from where I live), I toured it in my camper, visiting friends along the way.

Take time to consider what you might want to investigate. Anything goes! I've just sold a deer skin frame drum I made a few years ago because I want to buy a guitar. Take art classes, have a go on a potter's wheel, learn to play piano, join the choir, hire a camper van, explore a new area. Do whatever lights you up!

DON'T WAIT FOR RETIREMENT

I've been asked, more than once, what I would do if I only had six months left to live. Who would I call? Where would I visit? What burning thing would I do?

For years, my answer has always been the same: I would continue to live the way I do now. I've chosen not to wait for retirement to do all the things I've seen others put off until 'one day' or 'the right time'. Both my parents were diagnosed with life-changing illnesses in their early forties and they never got to do those things. In fact, my mum died when I was still in my twenties, so for me, that forever changed my view of 'the right time' to do anything.

From then on, I took courses, went on the trips, took risks...it was always there at the back of my mind, that I might not make it past fifty! In my early years, I lived more of a checklist 1) Visit New Zealand 2) Get a dog 3) Buy a campervan and travel. Now it's more a case of living in flow, seeing what resonates and letting my soul's whispers guide me.

When my budget was tight, I hiked locally, sleeping on airbeds on friends' floors. I planned travel around the cheapest train fares and borrowed friend's pets. I house sat, dog-walked and did everything I could to feel closer to my dreams.

Hold onto your dreams but hold them lightly. Allow them to evolve and adapt as you change. Take baby steps towards them, whenever you can. Be open to surprising opportunities, sometimes the most unexpected circumstances give us exactly what we need.

MAKE THE MOST OF EVERY MOMENT

I cried today. I was planning the decoration I would embroider onto my dear friend's funeral shroud. Not that she isn't alive and well, she's very healthy and vibrant but she's decided it's time to plan ahead.

I paused for a moment to wonder why I was crying. Partly because all her friends will be creating a thing of great beauty for her...then the next time we will see it, she'll be lying underneath it, awaiting her burial. I cried partly because I will miss her laughter and her wisdom terribly and I've had far too many final goodbyes in my life already, I'm never ready for another one.

And then I remembered. I have the gift of her life and her vitality right now and I can make the most of that. I can use my creativity to help create a thing of beauty and remembrance that will also be a legacy for her friends and family.

Death is never a final goodbye, just a parting of the ways until the next wondrous phase of whatever the Universe has in store for us.

The poignancy of someone reaching an age where they felt able to plan their own funeral definitely made me think about enjoying life and people now. So look up occasionally, enjoy the now and treasure all the people. None of us will be here forever.

YOU KNOW ALL THE ANSWERS

It's three a.m. I'm sitting on the kitchen floor in our studio apartment, I have a huge painting in front of me, half sun, half moon and I'm creating texture by free-flow writing over the paint. I'm asking myself "What shall I do? What do I need?".

I don't know what I'm writing but it's cathartic. It's a way to quieten my mind, distract myself from thought, to allow answers to arise from deep within me. By the time I'd finished writing, my answer was clear:

'Leave everything behind and go home'

I ended my relationship, quit my job and left London, to heal my heart, my body and my spirit. My then-boyfriend and I were renting an apartment in Docklands; our relationship had deteriorated rapidly, partly due to job stress, partly because he just couldn't 'hear' me.

I had so much going through my head I had difficulty sleeping, I would toss and turn for hours. At the time, I was doing an art journalling course on mandalas and decided to do the next chapter instead of lying in bed that night.

It's a writing technique, a form of automatic writing to just brain dump and it gets absorbed into the art. I'm not an artist as such, I'd always been told I was rubbish at art actually but this course helped me play with art creatively and intuitively.

When my brain won't switch off, I get my pens or paints out and just explore. Try it...get a journal or any paper you like; use pens, coloured pencils or paints and just play. Allow your subconscious mind to direct you, with words, patterns or designs. Maybe use your non-dominant hand to shift your perspective. Once the conscious part of your brain is quiet, the answers will come.

LET YOUR INNER CHILD OUT TO PLAY

My rescue pup will not do a wee in the garden if it's raining. So it's somewhat galling that her joy for walks overrides her desire to stay dry – she drags us both out for walks and we both have to get wet!

One day, it was too windy for an umbrella and my hood kept blowing off. To add insult to injury, I had drips of water going down my neck and splashing on my face. I was somewhat grumpy. She, on the other hand, excitedly dashed from one puddle to the next, tasting each one, heedless of the icy water. Suddenly she ducked her entire face right into a large muddy puddle, trying to pull something out.

When she couldn't quite get it, she bounced into the puddle, gleefully splashing and then looked outraged when a mini tidal wave of freezing water slopped over her back.

I couldn't help laughing, my mood lifted as I started splashing at the edges of her puddle with my boots. She was delighted that I joined in and soon we were both bouncing in and out of the pools of water, all grumpiness completely washed away, just abandoning ourselves to the joy of jumping in puddles.

My adult self didn't like wet weather but this was inner child-led! The child-like innocence of play is present in moments like that, those moments push us out of projections of dealing with wet muddy clothes, having to wash and dry the dog when we get back in, playing with Kali in that moment means I'm open!

Open to hearing birds sing, seeing blue sky and knowing the weather will clear later, I'm so much more present. Allow the child in you to lead the way sometimes; let her out, she's fun!

NOT EVERYONE WILL HEAR YOU AND THAT'S OK

I am staring at him in disbelief. Rage, frustration and utter hopelessness flooded me. We'd had yet another bust up, which led to yet another long drawn-out discussion about our needs, expectations, wants and desires.

And yet again, I believed we had finally reached a resolution, a way forward. This time I got him to write down his side of things and sign it. There it was, in black and white. No squirming out with "I don't remember saying that" or "You've twisted my words". To my horror, he still disowned what was right there in front of him.

It took me another couple of years and an ocean of tears before I finally came to the acceptance that there is absolutely nothing I can do to make another person truly hear me...not my tone of voice, the words I choose, my body language or my form of expression. And with that acceptance came a kind of peace. A deep inner calm that means I no longer fight or struggle to be heard. If someone can't or won't hear me, they're not my tribe and I don't waste energy trying to persuade them to see my point of view. It's so much easier now to recognise members of my tribe, the ones who have a similar level of acceptance; we hear each other without necessarily having to agree.

Don't waste time 'trying' to be heard, accept that not everyone will get you or understand your viewpoint and they don't have to for your perspective to be valid. Move on, others will find you and you will feel heard.

DIVORCE IS NOT FAILURE

We were sitting at a table in a crowded pub on the Isle of Wight on a Bank holiday weekend. We were both crying. We had finally agreed, together, that our marriage was over and that we would go our separate ways.

We had grown apart. We had very different views on what life should look like and how we should resolve the issues that arose between us. It was exhausting.

Divorce didn't mean I wasn't good enough or that I didn't try hard enough or even that I'll never get another chance. It means that I saw things differently than when we married. My values had changed. I'd lost myself within 'us' and I'd been battling to fight my back to myself.

My number one priority needed to be that I love myself first and foremost, to live in alignment with my core values and not to compromise in order to avoid conflict. I didn't really know that at the time though. All I knew, was that I was deeply unhappy. It took leaving and several years of deep inner work, to learn how to take responsibility for my own needs, wants and desires and how to articulate them clearly to another. Divorce is not a failure, it's growth and change and movement and it's absolutely ok.

SUICIDE COMES FROM AN ALTERED MIND STATE, DON'T BLAME YOURSELF

I was seventeen the first time I tried to commit suicide. After many years of sexual abuse, traumas, betrayals and feelings of utter hopelessness, of not belonging in this world, I'd reached the limit of my endurance. I was more afraid of living than of dying.

I've been back to that mind state many times over the years, each time believing there was no other way out. Over the decades, I slowly came to realise that these feelings were not permanent, they were transient. No matter how bad the situation, no matter how hopeless and helpless I felt, I can now see there was always a way forward.

Do not blame yourself if someone close to you took that path. There was nothing you could have said or done that would have changed things for them. I didn't reach out because I couldn't. It's highly likely they knew you were there, that you cared and it still didn't change a thing, because it was never about their relationship with you, it was only ever about the depth of pain they felt and could literally no longer live with.

Alena has dug deep to craft her chapter for you. She has had to overcome many wounds and says she is most inspired by women who live an authentic life and have healed from their past.

It's no surprise then, that she has done exactly that. A mother of two, her children, now grown-up, have been her guiding light in the toughest years.

She wrote her chapter to help support you in speaking your truth. She hopes her words give you hope on your darkest days.

@purebeingstudios

ALENA HAWK

BREAK THROUGH YOUR RESISTANCE TO CHANGE

I always dreamed of having a family and leading a 'normal' life where I grew up in Eastern Europe. However, the universe had different plans. By thirty, I emigrated to the UK with my husband, our baby girl and our three-year-old son. My husband was the only one of us who spoke English. It was such journey into the unknown! Growing up under a communist regime left me distrusting people's intentions, suspicious of their motives and unable to understand why they'd be kind to me.

Isolated and homesick, I hid behind a pushchair, speaking Czech so people wouldn't talk to me! I was mortified if anyone approached me and I lacked the confidence to learn English.

Fortunately, we had enough money for me to attend a language school and slowly, I began to overcome my fear of our new lifestyle. I'd felt terrible for leaving my parents, sister, niece and my friends in Europe. I held a belief that I'd only be happy if I lived like them, yet I'd made a very different choice for myself and I now see I was anxiously awaiting my parents' approval! It was difficult to be happy, knowing my parents weren't.

What I've learned is that it's ok to embrace your life choices without waiting for anyone's approval. I wish I'd known that happiness came in many different forms and that change is always inevitable, it's the only constant force in fact. Our personal growth and cultivation, in fact, depend on it. I now embrace my path and I embrace change, I look forward to meeting the next versions of myself.

DON'T GIVE UP HOPE...YOU CAN DO THIS!

I was officially homeless. I'd escaped an abusive marriage in the middle of the night with two children, nine and six years old. I'd fled to a friend's house. We had no belongings and our bank account was blocked.

After so much stress, it was wonderful to feel safe and able to sleep. I had a retail job and my own bank account but we were homeless for four months before we found a house...empty and dirty yet it was ours!

My friends were amazing, they kindly donated plates, bedding, mattresses and lots of other treasures. It was so important to me to believe that I would be able to build a new home for my children, I had to have faith in myself that I'd make this work without any support.

My friends played a significant part in this but equally, I knew I had to find the inner strength to do this. I never gave up hope of a better future for myself and my children. My children gave me a reason to get up every morning and we started rebuilding our lives as the three musketeers!

My learning is, if you're not dead, you can start over! You can absolutely rebuild your life from nothing. Things can be replaced. Emotional pain can be healed.

Darling, possessions and money mean nothing if you live in fear, if you don't feel safe or if your basic human needs aren't met. It is possible to walk through unpleasant darkness and find your light again.

LEARN TO TRUST THE FLOW, IT HAS YOUR BACK!

By thirty, I had a beautiful two-year-old son who was eagerly awaiting the arrival of his little sister. I had a reasonably good life in the country of my origin, we lived in an apartment in a small town. And I had my whole life planned out!

I planned on taking maternity leave after our baby arrived to help my husband with his business and I would visit my family every other weekend. None of that happened. In the spirit of a good wife, I followed my husband's crazy idea of moving across the world to start a new life. I had no idea what awaited me, I didn't speak English I had no idea how I would integrate! But integrate I did and I found so much out about myself in the process.

If I had chosen that safer option – my plan - and stayed with my parents in my country of origin, I would not know how strong I truly am. I wouldn't have learned about myself on the deepest of levels and I wouldn't have grown into my true authentic self.

By moving countries and trusting myself, I discovered my love for learning which has continued for the last twenty-four years and I learn everything in my second language, English!

I realised that very often, life had a better plan for me. I couldn't see it though while I was focusing on my parents beliefs and values and setting up my life, the way they lived theirs.

I now understand the importance of not fighting life and finding my flow.

You are SO worthy!

As I moved countries with my family, there were many challenges but what I hadn't foreseen was how quickly my relationship lost its balance. I couldn't work, which meant I lost my identity, my worth and my confidence and I allowed other people's emotions to overwhelm me. I remember praying for our family and our safety every single day. I was exhausted emotionally, mentally and physically. It took lots of effort just to exist actually.

I knew I needed to leave my marriage. I had nowhere to go back then and I didn't want to split the family but one day, my seven-year-old son asked me a very clear and direct question. I realised in that moment, that in trying to protect them, they were being affected as well as me.

This was a turning point in my life and still it took me another two years to get the courage to leave. As I look back on my life, I tell myself that I'm so worthy of being treated with respect, dignity and love. Getting back in touch with my true self and knowing my value took me years. Knowing my worth is an ongoing journey of self-love and I am finally learning to embrace my inwards journey.

My love...if you are reading this, this is your sign...you are worthy of a life you love. Just know that.

Look after yourself while you're grieving

I have lived through many things; one of the things I've lived through is my partner dying of suicide. When that happened, I simply froze. I was left with so many unanswered questions...my life felt like a movie. I couldn't relate to it. I found it so difficult to accept, that this was my and my children's reality.

My emotional pain was overwhelming and exhausting at every level and my body was physically in pain too. My brain froze and I went into surviving mode. I couldn't imagine anything more than getting through the next few minutes of my existence and finding my strength to do that was difficult.

One day my thirteen-year-old daughter gave me the greatest gift, she said "Mum, if you can't do this, neither can we!". I kind of 'woke up' from my pain and realised I had to help myself in order to help my children. I needed deep rest, I needed help.

Everyone's grief journey is such an individual and unique experience but I wish someone had told me to stop and take care of myself at the very beginning. Grief tends to come in waves but eventually, I learned to stand up. I'm able to meet the next waves of sadness or pain in grace now.

This precious life my love, is a mixture of happiness and sadness. Take care of yourself. Rest when you can, ask for help, allow your children to remind you, life is still here.

BRING RITUAL INTO YOUR LIFE

At the age of forty-five, I decided to become a yoga teacher. I wanted to learn about yoga philosophy (which resonated with me) and to gain more tools for my own healing.

When I went to the first training weekend, I asked my teacher what I could do with tension headaches. They were debilitating and frequent. "How can I make my body fitter, so I can move again?" was my next question.

She asked me gently, "Can you sit with yourself on this bolster and just breathe?". It was probably the most profound question someone had asked me in my entire life. I came from a place of pushing myself to perform, I wasn't respecting my body and I didn't understand that my body was telling me to pause. I didn't know it was ok to just take a breath and pause.

I had so much to do every single day, it was so difficult to pause and take time for myself. It was uncomfortable to stop and explore my stillness too. It was definitely a journey into the unknown parts of me. It required courage and compassion, much like everything else in life I've found.

So as a way of maintaining a balanced state, I started to allow myself to do my rituals and prayers, in order to show myself compassion. I'd practice the delicious art of restorative yoga most days and I've learned to accept that my yoga practice is a 'way of being' with myself, rather than simply doing and performing 'lots of poses' on my mat.

Think about starting a yoga practice to support the connection of your body, mind and breath. There are so many different styles of yoga to explore, find the one that suits your needs.

TRUST YOURSELF AND FOLLOW YOUR OWN WAY

There was a sense of relief and hope for me in the new beginnings I've created for my family but those new beginnings also brought doubt. I often doubted if I'd done the right thing and yet I somehow always trusted my instinct.

While I often didn't understand what lessons I was meant to be learning in my life...what I did believe in is that I am a spiritual being, having a human experience and that helped me to start trusting the process of life and trusting myself.

Trusting oneself and taking full responsibility for one's decisions is a journey. For me, it was a journey of connecting with my own intuitive process and knowing what I needed in order to heal. My ability to recognise my 'inner knowing' evolved into a greater trust in myself and it can for you too. Your inner knowing, your intuition, will be your guide, just do what you think is best and follow your own way.

LOVE YOUR SELF

I never really understood what self-love was. I spent most of my adult life looking outwards, serving others...looking after everyone else.

I willingly gave away my boundaries because I didn't love myself. I wish someone had told me that our adult life should start with the journey inwards, exploring oneself and knowing who we are.

A part of me used to worry that once I learned to 'see' myself, that I wouldn't be able to 'unsee' myself and that could be my greatest challenge. That hasn't been the case though. The process of personal growth has been and is a never-ending process. My journey so far has taught me that I'm not serving anyone well, if I don't serve myself first...simply as the old saying goes 'We can't pour from an empty cup'.

This also made me a question; 'How can I love another, if I truly don't love myself?'. It's why self-love and self-care starts with the 'Self'. I'm learning to acknowledge my Self more and more as I'm maturing. It took me a while to figure out that self-love comes from a greater sense of self-awareness and from that...self-acceptance.

From awareness comes choice. From choice comes integrity. From integrity comes self-acceptance and from self-acceptance comes a deep loving responsibility to keep choosing the path that leads us to our hearts and our most authentic selves.

Just in case you don't know, it is absolutely ok to recognise your needs before anyone else's and to act in a self-compassionate way. Start the day with a note to yourself: 'PS: I love you'.

A mother of two, Deborah says her children have been her biggest inspiration to finding her voice.

She has spoken up in her career, negotiated salaries and job terms, she's had to stand up for her medical choices and freedoms and she wrote her chapter in the hope that her words would resonate with another woman somewhere in the world, to encourage her to stand up for her own freedom too.

She says she hopes her reader can develop a 'feeling of belonging and acceptance of the many ways' we grow and learn as women.

@the_clary_sage

DEBORAH THOMAS HLADECEK

AGING IS A GIFT

Once I crossed the Rubicon of midlife, I began to accept myself. I let go of the fear of missing out or of letting others down. I realised the immense gratitude I had with age and the wisdom I'd acquired over the years. I didn't want to turn back, even if I could.

Some people never get the opportunity to grow old, as the Hindi adage goes, 'It's a privilege denied to many'. I feel that to curse aging is to dishonour those who departed this world without the sunspots and the crow's feet, without the self-confidence that takes years to attain.

With the physical signs of aging, also comes wisdom from the lessons learned, the love shared and the optimism of what each new day brought.

There were many people in my family that never got the opportunity to grow old and suffered many years with a genetic family illness. To have journeyed this far in life with my good health is something to be celebrated. It would seem disrespectful to my family to curse aging.

This life is the biggest gift.

TRY SOMETHING NEW

As an expat for fourteen years, I've explored new countries, cultures and food; currently I'm learning another language. I'm never far from doing something new, often out of necessity. It's challenging at times but does bring me happiness, a sense of novelty, accomplishment and growth. I've found that I get 'stuck in a rut' if I don't do new things now.

I used to find myself going through the motions of daily life: shopping at the same stores, driving the same routes, doing the same chores and visiting the same restaurants. Mostly because of the fear of living in a place that wasn't my homeland and lacking the familiarity of the culture I was raised in. But when I grew bored and thought I was unhappy in my new surroundings, I realised more doors were open to me, if I only had the courage to walk through them.

I sought out the company of friends who weren't afraid to try new things; some of them locals who would introduce me to new places and ideas. Connecting with people was my way out of the rut.

I find it's difficult to maintain an appreciative relationship with something that's always the same. I think as humans, we crave meaning! And for me, travelling, learning about different cultures, food, languages and learning new hobbies create joy. Scientifically, that's supported too as we create new neurons and neural pathways in our brains when we try new things.

Break routine, hack a habit and invest in something with real emotional value. Being on autopilot really trims away our joy and happiness. Try something new.

NEVER WALK PAST A PENNY

I don't remember where I learned this (probably from my dad) but I've done this for as long as I can remember, even when it felt embarrassing to do so! I have never walked past a penny on the ground without picking it up – even if it was dirty!

Maybe it was the proverb I learned as a child: 'Find a penny, pick it up, all day long you'll have good luck, pass that penny to a friend, your penny luck will never end'.

I'm a great believer in the law of attraction, so, when I say yes to even the smallest amount of value, I believe it sends a message to the Universe that I'm open to receiving any amount.

We live in a world that utilises money in exchange for goods and services, so, act in a manner that sends a clear message of your abundance mentality to the Universe! Pass that penny on to a friend as an act of good-will and you'll tell the Universe you even have enough to share.

Anecdotally, I can say that things worked out for me financially. While I never won the lottery, whenever I needed a financial boost the opportunity often presented itself. It was then up to me to recognise it and make those pennies shine, always passing some on to someone in need.

TAKE YOURSELF PAST COMFORT AND INTO THE WILD

While studying plant chemistry, I recognised something interesting about the wild lavender growing at high altitudes in Provence versus the iconic purple rows of cultivated lavender growing at lower elevations.

Wild lavender has a more varied chemical profile so it can survive storms and droughts or fight off invasive species, while cultivated plants in general, are nurtured, watered, weeded and have a predictable chemical profile consistent for suppliers. Cultivated plants are coddled, whereas wild plants are resilient and adaptive to stress.

I feel I've had a coddled life in that way; my body has expected regular meals, warm showers and a bed...a sense of safety. I've come to realise though, that if we don't put our bodies and minds in positions where we need to adapt, we'll have difficulty coping with stress; we're simply not practiced at it.

One day, I thought I could tolerate a bit of a cold rinse after my warm shower. So, I tried it for one minute. I felt so good afterwards, I increased it to three minutes.

I also decided to try intermittent fasting. I decided to push myself past breakfast with only a herbal tea, then I'd have a big lunch that I appreciated even more. I began to feel exhilarated by restraint in certain areas and grateful for what followed afterwards.

I feel more resilient, stronger and appreciative now that I take those cold showers, when I fast or push myself physically in the elements. Try taking yourself past comfort and into the wild sometimes. You'll strengthen your inner reserves and you might just gain confidence, become more creative and have some rewarding experiences.

TUNE INTO NATURE RATHER THAN THE CALENDAR

I used to make New Year's resolutions to start new projects, exercise routines or nutritional cleanses but I'd often fail and I couldn't understand why, as I'm a very motivated person.

Later in life, after learning that my biological grandfather was Irish, I learned more about his culture, watching Celtic ancestral wisdom podcasts and reading about the Celtic wheel of the year. That learning was so different to how I grew up in New England, USA with the four seasons. Nowadays, I'm an aromatherapist also studying astro-herbalism, so I resonate with the periods of planting, pruning and harvesting as per Celtic tradition and the moon phases.

The more I got in touch with nature, especially in my own garden, tuning into her rhythms and cycles, I began to understand that January 1st was just a calendar date set by man in the beginning weeks of winter in the northern hemisphere!

During those short days, I noticed my instincts were to conserve energy, to hibernate so to speak. Naturally, I feel like this is a time to settle in with my family, to bake, do crafts – make a mess; not to begin a fitness routine, clean the house or start new projects. The right time for those things for me, is in March when my feelings, desires and motivations begin to instinctively bloom with the golden optimism of the daffodils and crocuses of springtime. Nature is a wise teacher.

Next time you feel you should do something, ask yourself how you feel when you think about doing it...line up with your natural inclinations and your motivation will be there, regardless of what the calendar tells you.

DON'T GO TO BED ANGRY

When I began dating my husband, we made a pact to never go to bed angry. We made the pact, after we'd done just that! We'd both got the worst night's sleep, tossing and turning, rehashing the argument in our minds. We agreed that some sort of resolution should happen before nightfall, so that the next day we could begin to assess the argument and speak with more lucidity and kindness.

We have since extended this to our children too. Never go to bed angry with your spouse, partner, child, roommate or parents. If an argument hasn't come to a resolution by bedtime, we call a truce, apologise for the argument - not an admission of any wrongdoing but we agree to discuss it further in the morning, after a good night's sleep. Mornings bring fresh perspectives.

Bringing anger into our place of rest and rejuvenation, into our dreamworld where our physical and spiritual bodies are meant to heal, isn't good for anyone. Resolution comes easier when we diffuse the anger before bedtime. A couple of ways we do this is to say, "I'm sorry for my part in this" and a physical hug - heart to heart - helps us to calm down and reset high emotions.

This has been such a relief; we always feel so much lighter when our heads hit the pillow.

BE INTERESTED IN WHAT INTERESTS YOUR CHILD

When my children were young and had a range of interests that weren't necessarily interesting to me, I made a conscious choice to really listen and take an interest in them. I could name my son's favourite Pokémon. I indulged in his ideas of superhero mashups and would ask questions about whose powers were better.

When my daughter collected rocks and crystals, I surprised her with a little shelf to display them, even though to me they were just ordinary rocks. When she loved baking, I'd buy ingredients and decorations for her, too. Our children need to be seen and feel confident, in who they're becoming. For me, my job as a mother was to support them in all their new and unfolding interests. They looked to me for approval and I never wanted to stifle their creativity or fascinations.

The hidden benefit now they're teenagers, is that I've laid down the groundwork for trust as they built their confidence. They talk openly with me about topics I never would have talked to my parents about. While I didn't have the bandwidth to engage in every new interest my children had, I did find meaningful areas to really connect with them and I'm so pleased I did. This is also an on-going engagement as I continue to find those data points of connection with their new and developing interests. I feel this can happen at any stage in a relationship and in all types of relationships.

GROW SOMETHING

In kindergarten, we planted seeds into little cups filled with earth. Watering them, we placed them on the classroom windowsill and watched them grow. Each day, we eagerly checked on them, waiting for them to push through the soil. There was much wonder and amazement – and optimism.

Over the years, in my lowest and darkest moments, I've found that seeing something grow in my garden has brought me hope. Watching the seasons change, going through her cycles of birth, blossoming, death and re-birth, unaware of the dramas going on with me or the world, has reminded me that seeds too, grow in the dark but eventually bloom.

I'm an herbalist and backyard gardener, so I encourage everyone to grow something. When you do that, you're declaring to yourself that there will be a
tomorrow.

Spiritually, growing plants also supports the root chakra, so planting grounds me and I feel a sense of belonging. When my perennial plants come back each year, I'm reminded that the world is still spinning and I'm still here, no matter where I live.

If you're feeling lost or losing hope, try taking a moment to be in nature, to witness what's growing around you. I find just focusing on one plant or just one flower and putting my attention on it completely, gets me out of my own way and regenerates my spirit.

Sumi has spent her whole career as a doctor dedicated to the care of her patients.

Her father inspired her to use her voice on behalf of those who couldn't speak for themselves. She says it's been an honour to work as a doctor and now she is using her voice to speak her wisdom in other areas of her life, including writing this beautiful chapter.

She hopes her stories inspire and help you. That has always been her life's purpose and now her words in this book impact women on a much wider scale!

@dr_chatterjee_ncimhealthcare

SUMI CHATTERJEE

MEDITATION WILL HELP YOU HEAR YOUR TRUE SELF

According to Sigmund Freud, the ego is a component of our personality. It is said to develop from our identity, it's how we perceive ourselves. It is said that when we're children, around the age of seven years old, we start to stand alone from being one with our mother. We begin to become an individual.

As such, the ego keeps our focus on 'I'. I remember as a teenager thinking, 'no-one has ever experienced love like me', 'no-one has ever experienced heart break like me'...the endless cycles of the ego's reverence for me was on repeat, looping through the generational vortex, I now understand that it's a completely normal process and necessary part of growing up.

I appreciate all these years later, that my ego has been my silent nemesis, compulsively making me use my mind to justify its biases whether individual or at a collective level.

In my experience, the practice of meditation has meant I've learned to question the 'ego-mind'. It's where I'm found stillness to hear my true Self. I believe it's our true Self that is actually 'united consciousness'.

For me, it's the only true basis for harmony, happiness and societal peace. When I look beyond the ego, to the real source of a collective consciousness, I see the inner light of all our beings.

Overcoming the ego has taken work, I had to adopt a beginner's mindset. The philosopher Epictetus said that if we let the ego tell us that we have arrived and have figured it all out, it prevents us from learning further, that we need to broaden our minds, read books, keep learning and remind ourselves of how much we don't know, in other words, to remain humble.

All that is precious and beautiful within me, honours all that is precious and beautiful within you.

You and I, are one.

NOTICE THE SIGNIFICANT AND THE INSIGNIFICANT

My dad once described to me how vast the universe was, so vast in fact that the size of our earth seemed almost insignificant, maybe the size of a dust particle at best. That totally blew my mind, how our human race pales into insignificance, how WE can pale into insignificance!

I felt insignificant at school, the last one standing, not yet picked to play a team sport. I felt insignificant working in a large institution, I felt insignificant when my friend was chatted up and I was ignored, it all mattered to me.

I did however, place huge significance on my education to become a doctor, it was my father's dream not mine, I remained in denial; qualifying as a doctor was my end goal. Once achieved, I was lost, my personality hugely mismatched with such a responsible career, I lived in constant anxiety and fear. In hindsight, if I'd had a chance to visit my younger self, I would have told her not to get too caught up in either the huge significance of things or the insignificance I often felt.

I have found the need to surrender to the process of life rather than fight it, maintaining the significance of stillness, in the insignificance of life's events.

Remember precious one, you are significant to your family, friends and this world. Have an awareness of when you place huge significance on something that may be stressing you out: breathe, journal, colour, do yoga...whatever you need, in order to transform your stress to calm, so you can see the bigger picture.

MEDITATE FOR A CALM MIND

With chaos around me, meditation created the calm. I first experienced the power of meditation whilst lying in 'corpse pose' at the end of a yoga class, just noticing my breath cultivated a serenity within me. Suddenly the past and future (where my mind spent most of its time) fell away, giving me a peaceful transcendence.

Over time, the little meditation I did slipped away as work became increasingly time pressured and I became overwhelmed with stress. One day after seeing nearly thirty patients and then doing endless paper work, I broke down in tears. I felt underappreciated, overworked, all autonomy was lost, so much so that I wanted to end my life.

Instinctively I knew if I carried on like this, cancer would visit me and it did. I often wonder if I manifested it out of distress, the divine feminine trapped within me. Following surgery, a charity gifted me with an eight-week 'mindfulness-based stress reduction' course, a form of meditation. It transformed my healing.

It helped me to create a daily mediation practice. I have learned that, as well as the calming effects of meditation, it also affects genes. We all have telomeres, they are found at the end of chromosomes (like the caps at the end of shoe laces). Their job is to protect our DNA. Research has proven that three months of daily meditation lengthens those telomeres and that, in turn, has positive effects on longevity and disease.

Be kind to yourself; anyone can meditate. Create a regular practice and watch the magic unfold.

In moments of overwhelm, BREATHE...

The breath whispers in my ear, 'I will stand by you for all your life, meditate with me and find your light'

The breath is with us from the moment we're born to our very last breath, our deepest friend, a golden thread running through the tapestry of our lives. Always there to change its rhythm and pace, mirroring our emotions, the big sighs of relief, the breaths we hold because of tension and the overwhelming gasp of wonder to an ethereal vision.

We often don't appreciate the authenticity of its being. I was an anxious child fearful of going to school, I would breathe so fast that I made myself dizzy and my little heart would race so quickly. They had to give me medication to keep it under control. Now I'm grown up, I understand it's the body's natural reaction to fear and stress. I've learnt to soothe my anxious child with a breath charm. Just breathe deep and slow and let the magic happen.

I breathe to calm myself. In for six, out for four. Inhale...one...two...three...four, exhale one...two...three... four... five...six. Keep going, honour your breath with your heart and soul.

Death is not the end

'Why weep my love, death is timelessness'

I have a saying 'as soon as we are born, we are dying'. The body is programmed to grow, reproduce and die. It's a simple fact of nature. So, I believe we have to make the most of the gift of life. I speak from a place of glimpsing the other side.

A few years ago, I was dying. In that experience, I had the most incredible odyssey, I was at the interface of life and death and I could see the other side. I saw a vortex of light with shimmering gold, I felt there were spirits who had once lived, inviting me to step over into the orb of golden light and I was tempted. But something pulled me back.

I feel so honoured to have experienced that and ever since, I've realised that death is actually not the end but merely a transition to a place of serenity and immortality.

Don't deny yourself music

'Music - life's poetry in song, without it, life is barren, cold and forlorn'

I used to be a DJ. Music was the backdrop of my life, holding the keys to the thousands of memories in my timeline. Without it, I wouldn't be here, it let me release so much as a child, from unrequited love and being bullied to arguments at home. I felt suicidal but music swept me up to heaven above, giving me peace and love.

Music seems to remain the lifeblood of the young, shaping the fashions and attitude of the newly sprung. And when we unite, music has a magical power to shoot moonbeams from our fingers. Invincible and strong, we express what we couldn't before through tears, laughter and words in songs. I keep those stories close to my heart when I feel lost in times of sorrow and falling apart.

The bedrock of connectedness, music unifies, through history its effects ripple through from sermon to tribal song. Songs of a revolution, articulating the essence of love, religious ceremonies, hymns, sound healing and mantras from above. Don't deny yourself the music, it is your life's song.

Travel...let it be your soothing balm

'Travel is fatal to prejudice, bigotry and narrow mindedness
and many of our people need it sorely on these accounts'
Mark Twain

I'm speechless when I travel and full of endless speech when I return. My dream was to be an airhostess, instead I had an arranged marriage with science and medicine, the inadvertent bride to a subject that felt beyond me.

Travel was my true love. Whenever I was released from the shackles of ancestral expectation, I would soar high like a phoenix rising from the ashes and landing back in her arms. To feel the tropical rain on my skin, the beat of the humming bird's wings in all its shimmering green plumage, the sacred Tibetan sky burial and Saturn with its rings seen through a ginormous telescope in Chilean skies.

I loved my animal encounters from Alaskan bears to African elephants, Indian tigers and the spectacular iridescence of fish swimming amongst the colourful coral. My favourite memory, pelican sunrise at Monkey Mia the Australian west coast.

One of the best days of my life, I had an early morning encounter with pelicans arriving on the beach while I was waiting to see the dolphins...just the Pelicans and me, my most intimate encounter with nature imprinted in my life's memoir.

Live your life now, have no regrets, don't wait, I am full of gratitude for all I have seen, it has been the most soothing balm.

ALWAYS HAVE HOPE

Hope, is a light that never goes out,
an angel embracing you with pure love.

I believe that without having hope, I would already be dead. I was admitted to hospital a few years back, I had fallen ill. Profound nausea and dizziness, unable to eat, drink, I knew then I was dying. Emergency fluids and urgent scans of my body were initiated. I was told the unthinkable, my breast cancer from years past (which had been in remission) had spread everywhere, to my brain, lungs, kidneys and spine.

From then on, I was labelled with 'Do not resuscitate' and the 'End of life' palliative care pathway was placed into motion. But I didn't feel my death was imminently inevitable.

I had faith, the love of my friends and family surrounding me and in a little corner was 'hope' standing her ground. Stoking up my dying coals with a fire of infinite possibility, hope revealed a path less travelled... overgrown thorned bushes and a single white rose.

Closing my eyes, I trusted the process. Locked in a healing tomb of radiotherapy and prayers hoping for the enlightenment I sought, 'Please just let me live again' and I did. Hope really does bring dreams to life, always have hope.

The nurturing love and encouragement from her mystic soul sisters, her Daoist siblings and her interfaith family, supports Deborah to give voice to that which is hers to be expressed.

She felt a deep inner calling to join this book collaboration and trusts that Spirit will guide her chapter into the awareness of those who need it most.

She invites readers to glean their own unique interpretations and meanings from her words, trusting them to hold close what resonates and release what doesn't.

@revdebart

REV. DEB CONNOR LI XIAO YI 笑意

SPIRITUAL GUIDANCE ISN'T ALWAYS SENT VIA A CHOIR OF ANGELS

One day while walking my beloved greyhounds, one of them did her business literally right next to the dog poo bin... handy!

I bagged it up and dropped it in bin. A thought occurred: If I'm going to pick up someone else's crap, even if I do it with love, I'd best be willing (and able) to drop it at the first opportunity before the stink sticks. Spiritual guidance with a practical message delivered on a dog walk.

I love this moment for so many reasons. A prompt to be mindful of what I pick up and how long I carry it. And a reminder that spiritual guidance isn't always delivered by a choir of angels singing hallelujah as they hand over a neatly written scroll.

Guidance is everywhere, if we choose to see it.

USE AN ANALOGY TO HELP YOU UNDERSTAND YOUR RESPONSES

'Sometimes I'm a trampoline, sometimes I'm a wine glass'

I remember first using this analogy when I was facilitating a group coaching session: it resonated deeply with people.

I don't always remember the specific incidents in my life that led me down particular thought paths. But remembering the allegories, stories, poems and descriptive parallels I create to represent the embodied learning – that I find much more powerful and memorable.

Appreciating my varied responses in life requires my understanding of my stable consistency. The consistency is 'me'. I am the consistent part of any life equation. That doesn't mean I need to respond consistently in every situation. So sometimes I'm a trampoline and sometimes I'm a wine glass. And that's okay. The analogy vividly demonstrates why some things shake off effortlessly whilst others affect me so deeply I can barely function.

Imagine pouring red wine into a glass. The glass easily holds the wine and any stains on the glass quickly rinse away under a running tap. Now imagine pouring the same wine onto a trampoline, the wine runs through the webbing, leaving it stained even after washing. The trampoline could feel inadequate for its inability to hold wine.

Throw a house brick onto that same trampoline and it absorbs the impact, stretches, then rebounds immediately, impressively bouncing the brick away. Throw that brick onto the wine glass and the glass shatters irreparably, leaving behind a feeling of inadequacy and brokenness.

Creating descriptive analogies has helped align me to my life purpose – I understand my strengths and challenges, I know when to ask for help and I accept my capacities and limitations while making sense of my world. We all respond individually to life's fluctuations, with different feelings, emotions and physiological responses. We are beautifully unique. Each day we are different, changed by our experiences of the day before. Our movement through life's stages shapes us and sometimes destabilises us.

We are fabulously human: we don't always navigate life easily and yet we can still make it through the unpredictability. What we do in the moment may not be the best we are capable of in life – but if that's all we can manage in the moment, it is enough.

We are all human, let's go easy on ourselves and each other.

STUDYING AN ANCIENT TEXT CAN BRING YOU PEACE, STILLNESS AND DEEPER INSIGHTS

I cannot overstate the value of choosing an ancient text that calls to you and studying it deeply. I have been exploring the Dàodé jīng 道德經 for two decades now.

For me the essence of studying the text deeply has been about understanding not just the superficial meaning but also its context, political background, cultural influence, as well as its practical wisdom in today's world, in my own life. Summarising the eighty-one chapters of the Dàodé jīng into one hundred one-liners of wisdom helped me to identify what truly resonated with me.

Deep contemplation of this text has shaped my view of the world, my ability to stand back and let things be and to practise its teachings in my day-to-day life. Result: a deeper understanding of my own self.

Without any pre-existing skills in the original language, I have lovingly undertaken a character-by-character translation of my chosen text. Although arduous at times this process enriched my understanding and changed my perspective. Sitting with this text consistently as a spiritual practice I have at last completed my own heartfelt translation in words and art for a book soon to be published.

Coming to a spiritual text over and over again – going to its source to embody its wisdom – can shape how we live our lives, how we feel about ourselves and our place in the world.

Studying a spiritual work does not need to be academic. Show up consistently to your chosen text, read a paragraph, then sit and allow those words to infuse inside you: without analysis, simply sit with it. Your Heart will absorb the meaning if you take your head out of the way.

FOOD ADDICTION IS A THING: YOU ARE NOT ALONE

I remember the day I found out that food addiction was actually a thing. It was also the day I realised that I wasn't weak or useless and I wasn't the only one who experienced the phenomenon of feeling compelled to eat.

What relief! The insanity and utter despair of sitting crying on my kitchen floor putting bread into my mouth that I didn't want to eat. I couldn't understand my own behaviour. But trying to fathom the unfathomable was a waste of time and energy.

Behaviour change through creative transformation developed my understanding that addiction is a spirit level malady requiring a creative spiritual solution. My journey from food addiction to food sobriety would take up an entire book. In short, I identified my triggers – foods that if I started eating I couldn't stop: for me they were sugar, alcohol, wheat, caffeine and dairy. I made daily spiritual practice non-negotiable. Using creativity to go deep into my spirituality was a game-changer. The compulsion to overeat left me at the same time an artist burst out of me. I may have been an overeater on the outside but inside I was a starving artist.

Now art is how I pray. Art is my meditation practice. Creativity holds me in a way that does not depend on results. The creative process nourishes me. This creative sustenance sees me through the worst of times and the best of times – without judgement.

If you recognise addiction in your own life – food, TV, work, social media, relationships, shopping, alcohol or anything you go to for comfort or to 'numb out' – know that you are not alone, you are not broken. Support is available and you can navigate through addiction to a life of recovery.

I promise you that living in recovery is well worth the journey. Take your first step towards recovery today – your future self will thank you.

CONSIDER HOW YOU SAY 'THANKS'

I don't remember exactly what I was doing when this insight landed, likely in one of my more reflective slowing down, pausing, observant moments. I suddenly realised how pointless my use of the word 'thanks' had become. An English pleasantry I tossed in someone's direction without any genuine sentiment.

I resolved to replace that throwaway word with a heartfelt 'thank you'. While it never felt strange to stop and reflect on whether I was actually thankful to a person, it did feel rather 'old school' to say 'thank you' or 'thank you so much'. This expression of genuine conscious gratitude shifted my energy and changed my outlook.

Now when I thank someone – a bus driver, retail worker, restaurant staff, a friend, anyone – I first check with myself for feelings of real gratitude. Initially I needed to dig deep to summon up a genuine feeling of thankfulness: only then would I look the person in the eye and say an honest 'thank you'.

This simple practice has enhanced my connections to others, deepened my gratitude practice, and increased my awareness of what I'm truly thankful for. So, when I say thank you for reading this, I really mean THANK YOU from the Heart and Soul of me: thank you so much.

FIND A TOOL FOR SPIRITUAL GROWTH THAT RESONATES WITH YOU

There are many tools for personal development and spiritual growth. One of my favourites is the enneagram, an ancient wisdom system describing nine personality types or 'operating systems'. We each have all nine inside us with one that dominates. That 'type' is how we meet and greet our world, how we understand and operate, where we get our energy from, what our fears and drivers are.

Seeing myself and others through the lens of the enneagram has allowed me to let go of judgment: to meet myself and others as they are, rather than how I would have them be. Appreciating how each of the nine types views, experiences and operates in the world increases my capacity for empathy and compassion.

As an enthusiastic type seven living with a peace-making type nine husband, I now understand his silence as giving space for me to speak rather than apparent indifference. Just one of the ways the enneagram has enhanced our relationship.

Through enneagram wisdom I easily identify when I am operating – personally and spiritually – in healthy ways that allow me to live authentically in the world. I am able to quickly identify any unhealthy functioning and adjust my path. The enneagram resonates deeply with me and applying its principles helps my real Self show up as a Presence of Love in the world.

Having a useable tool for personal development and spiritual growth may not smooth out all the bumps in the road, but it will give you a framework to lean into for self-cultivation: a place to find companionship and support from others using that system.

Whether it's the enneagram or any other tool for growth, be open to finding a system you can work with long term, one that deeply resonates with your own inner wisdom. Find something that doesn't put you in a box – look for a tool that shows you the box... and how to get out of it.

PAINT TO REFRAME OLD NARRATIVES

At the age of forty-nine I felt called to gather some art supplies and visit Morocco – somewhat surprising as I wasn't an artist back then. Spirit woke me one night at three in the morning under a bright Moroccan moon and my spiritual assignment was delivered: get up and create!

Despite initial resistance creativity became my daily spiritual practice. In committing to this practice I found my authentic Self, a connection with the Divine and the world around me to a depth I previously could not have imagined. I believe creativity IS spirituality: lean into one to find the other.

Art is the vehicle through which the Universe speaks to me. Over time I have developed a variety of writing, painting and creative practices that serve specific purposes on my spiritual quest. One such practice is to paint a canvas that represents a narrative I wish to reframe, a story I repeatedly tell myself and want to let go of. This painting is purely for me to express my current narrative: no one else will see it, so it only needs to make sense to me. It doesn't need to look pretty or skilful, just real and honest.

 Once the painting is dry, I thank it for being the visual representation of the story I wish to reframe before painting over the entire canvas in a single colour. I then allow myself to be guided to areas of the still wet paint and scrape these off, revealing parts of the original beneath. I feel this symbolises moving on from the old narrative while taking useful learning and experiences with me. A gentle and deeply transformative practice that doesn't require analytical thought or artistic skill.

The best way to appreciate this embodied practice is by trying it. Grab a canvas and some acrylic paints – the easiest medium to work with for this process. Choose colours that represent your current narrative and get them on the canvas, using your hands, brushes, a spoon, anything: simple blobs of paint, abstract, figurative – create whatever feels meaningful to you.

When its dry, choose a colour to overpaint with – you'll find darker colours work best. Set your intention to reframe your old narrative and cover your entire painting, then scrape back some areas allowing your original to show through.

Trust this transformational exercise, let go of overthinking and allow the painting process to gently reframe your internal dialogue.

DISSOLVING THE DITCH OF YOUR OWN CREATION

 Rather than hold onto unhelpful narratives I like to create descriptive analogies to represent the lessons learned. One such analogy is 'dissolving the ditch of my own creation'.

In past moments of despair and hopelessness I have felt like I'm stuck in a ditch. Thinking about how I ended up in the ditch, rather than focusing solely on the misery of the ditch itself, helped me find a practical way up and out.

Although sometimes difficult to accept, acknowledgement of my own contribution to creating the ditch is a must if I want to move forward. I need time deep in my emotional ditch, as long as it takes, to explore and understand it – to do my own 'inner ditch' work.

If someone – however well-meaning – pulls me out, the ditch is still there and I can fall back into it. While offering me a ladder or a rope may help me climb out, the ditch is always there waiting for me. The only way that truly works for me is to dissolve the ditch.

Examining, understanding and being in that ditch may need support from trusted friends, a therapist or spiritual guide. In dissolving the ditch, I liberate myself. I am free! For sure I'll create another ditch, that's part of life's experience: I repeat the process, remember the new learning and let go of old narratives.

Being 'ditch-bound' can feel like the end of the world. Reach out for support when you need to. Take breaks and rest from the process of the inner healing work. Continue when you feel ready.

Know that you are held with loving energetic support by myself and every woman contributing to this book. You are not alone.

You are held with loving energetic support by every woman in this book...
we wrote it for you.

A single mum, a leader and a mentor, Kerry has been drawn to several female spiritual teachers in the last few years, all of whom have inspired her to use her voice more and more.

She resonated with the call-out for women to write this book, she says the words 'sang to her', she recognised herself in them and followed her intuition.

Her hope is that in reading her words, you come to know the goddess you truly are and follow your own intuition.

@kerry_walton222

KERRY WALTON

A LOVE LETTER TO WOMEN

Growing up I was surrounded by wonderfully strong, yet gentle women with the most generous of hearts. Nothing has compared to the nurturing and nourishment I have received from women over the years, I don't think I ever fully appreciated just how fucking amazing they were until much later in life.

I have cherished friendships from when I was just a tot, that have survived the years, others have formed recently, yet we feel like we've known each other for millennia.

My female friends are my life support, my soul sisters, mothers by proxy...they've turned up with flowers because they want to share the beauty of them, they've held me when tears have threatened to overpower me and they never questioned my inability to explain why.

There are moments with them that make me laugh to the point of almost wetting myself...glorious deep belly laughing that reverberates in the body and keeps me lifted for days. They've played match makers (one actually resulted in a marriage, the other in a tale that still keeps us entertained!). They know where my scars have come from, some of them were there to witness the wounds being made and some were there to kiss them better.

We hold space for each other and love each other and those feelings ripple out beyond my immediate circle and into my desire to support and champion other women. I want to lift them, to tell them it's okay to have something to say and to want to use their voices, I want them to do things on their terms, to be seen, understood and accepted.

You are as magnificent as you always dreamed you could be...and that's something we should celebrate, revelling in our respective radiance and coming together rather than being pitted against each other. If you're already blessed to have women in your life, don't let too much of life or 'being too busy' get in the way of spending soul enriching time with them.

If this hasn't been your experience of other women or female energy so far...give it another chance...dare to be vulnerable in the company of other women and I promise the rewards will be worth it.

ACCEPT AND SURRENDER, THEN DO IT A BIT MORE....

The trick I find, is actually knowing when to let go. It's all about releasing the reins and falling into a state of trust, that it's all going to be ok, opening yourself up to being vulnerable (which is an absolute strength!), handing over control to something bigger than you and believing it will all work out for your highest good...whatever that may look like.

I'm absolutely a work in progress with this one; it certainly doesn't come naturally for me; in fact its counter intuitive to the way I'm wired but I have come to recognise it as being the complete truth. When I surrender, things just seem to flow and magnetise towards me.

Planning is good but there comes a point where certain aspects are beyond my control and rather than grasping or torturing myself about how things are going to work out, I accept where I'm at and surrender, releasing my desires and intentions into the Universe, sitting back and expecting miracles.

A wonderful saying I picked up from someone recently was: 'Accept what is, let go of what was and have faith in what will be'. Be present, live with and in the 'now'. Accept and surrender.

DATING POST FIFTY...RETAIN YOUR SENSE OF HUMOUR!

When I first went onto a dating app, I put my profile live and literally suspended it within minutes...it would have been seconds but I couldn't find the 'suspend profile' button!

Honestly, I felt like a prize cow being put on show and led around the auction ring. I felt so exposed, I was just on my journey back from the breakdown of a long-term relationship, getting back to a healthy level of self-esteem but I tried again.

And...there is strangeness out there! People who clearly lack emotional intelligence, some carry baggage and just want to dump it on someone, it opened my eyes (to some things I'd rather not see again!) but I also met some lovely people.

Overall it's been a positive experience. My chats with one guy were sexually charged and incredibly liberating, I closed it down without meeting up in the end (I doubt I could have got myself into some of the positions he wanted to put me in!). And a few people later, came Mr Lovely. I think I fell a little in love with him on our first date but it turns out he had to prioritise his 'cause' and 'change the world'....sigh...

If you're wondering whether to use an app, just retain your sense of humour, hold it all lightly, know what you want and more importantly what you don't. Honour all your boundaries and just be yourself.

Beyond anything though, know that you're already enough. Unaccompanied, solo but certainly not less than. Focus on loving yourself fully so that evolving with another human is simply a bonus. If you can truly know yourself before bringing your 'whole' self/wholeness into a relationship, it means you're not looking for someone else to complete you. You already are.

WHEN THEY LEAVE HOME

When my son was due to leave home for university, in amongst the logistics of last-minute student details, I got busy having a total meltdown. I panicked that time had finally run out for me to give him the tools he'd need to survive, let alone thrive. "He doesn't even know how to make a cheese sauce...what sort of mother am I?" I shared with my coach.

I genuinely felt like I'd failed him because I hadn't equipped him with the ability to 'throw something together' from the fridge.

She asked me "What's the best thing about him?". I felt my face soften and an enormous smile form, tears sprang. I replied "He gives the best hugs". That changed my perspective in an instant. In my heart, I knew I'd done good. I was sending a wonderful affectionate, emotionally intelligent human out into the world, the rest was up to him.

I had identified myself by being 'mum'. It was hard to even know who I was when he went. If this is you, find yourself again, reclaim the space they resided in. Spread out into their room, use the space to display beautiful pieces of art, go there just to play music that moves you, dance there!

Remember how good it feels to be alive, embrace the change that their leaving brings. You have new adventures to live with your accumulated wisdom and experience. Make a list called 'How to live the fuck out of my life' and get busy ticking things off it!

LET GRIEF FLOW THROUGH YOU

I kissed her so gently on the cheek and whispered in her ear, "You can go now Mum". Those who could be there, were sitting around her hospital bed, others said their goodbyes over the phone while we held the receiver to her ear.

I think she heard us. I hoped she could feel the love in the room...and then I sensed the energy leave her. My beautiful mum had passed to spirit.

Weeks away from her seventieth birthday, she was taken by that shitty ovarian cancer that we didn't even know existed inside her until two weeks before.

No-one can ever prepare for grief. It can bring you to your knees. I remember finding myself on the kitchen floor many times in the months that followed, crying relentless big horrible tears that dragged my waterproof mascara down my face. I sobbed to the point of nearly retching, the physical pain was so great. And then it would pass, if I allowed it. If I accepted it as an emotion, it would flow through and on. It could be replaced by another, even laughter. Feel it all. Don't shy away from the pain and let it go when it subsides, allow it to be replaced by whatever wants to come next. Don't try to hold it...it's all ok.

MAINTAIN A BOND WITH YOUR EX, YOUR CHILDREN ARE YOUR COMPASS

Even now, I'm not sure where the words actually came from. Certainly, I hadn't rehearsed them. I didn't even know the thought behind them existed until that very moment and if I'd have stopped to check myself or think about it, even for just a second, I don't think I'd have ever said it.

But once the words were out, I knew to my very core I'd spoken the truth...our marriage was over. Endings are hard, especially if you still love the person you're parting from but that doesn't mean it's not right to leave. I carried a lot of guilt for a long time for being the one to voice things out loud but I've since offered myself forgiveness because it was exactly what we both needed, what our family needed, what was right for our son.

And next came all the messiness that separation and ultimately divorce brings with it. We worked together to salvage a relationship that meant we could co-parent our son from separate places and somehow, in doing so, we ultimately developed a far greater bond than we'd ever had before.

Not straight away no and not without some pretty challenging times where egos, past hurts or new partners threatened to undermine it but we endured. At the heart of all we faced, was the love we both felt for our son. He started as and has remained, our absolute priority. His welfare was our compass.

For me, every decision I made came from a place of love - for my son, myself or my ex-husband. That helped me heal and it guided me, seeing me through the toughest of situations. I let my heart lead the way, rather than my pain or my ego or other people's opinion. Now we're blessed with a gorgeous grown-up son who can express himself openly and my ex-husband remains one of my closest friends.

If this situation and my experience speaks to you, be kind to yourself. Find what's true for you and trust you can navigate your way through the chaos, pain, sadness, hurt or anger all of the above! Find your compass and follow it.

MAKE A CONNECTION WITH PEOPLE, EVEN STRANGERS

I used to cringe when my mum would do it. She'd spark up a conversation from nowhere with a complete stranger, just randomly and it seemed so effortless! We could be on a bus, waiting on a cold platform at a train station, in a shop...anywhere!

And they'd warm to her, immediately. You'd see their faces light up in response to her attention and I was both envious and embarrassed in equal measure.

Years later I find myself doing the exact same thing without aspiring to it or even thinking about it much. I seem to have taken on her mantle!

Connection with another human is visceral. I feel an overriding need to witness other people, acknowledge them, connect with them, for me, it's a physical thing. If I deliberately don't connect with someone after knowing I've been 'called' to, the feeling of having 'missed' something important stays with me, it lingers and I won't settle.

Never underestimate the power a simple smile can have. A moment of connection can literally lift a person's energy and change the course of their day (dare I say their life – who knows!) you never know what the impact will be!

YOU'LL FIND YOUR TRIBE

"You'll never get a bloke if you talk like that!" was the honest, supposed supportive response of my friend's husband during a late-night conversation about life, beliefs and finding me a partner. For once, maybe for the first time ever, I'd been totally honest, spilling my truth about how I really felt, being a part of something much bigger, connected to everything and everyone, souls having a human experience, here to learn and love etc and it seems I completely blew his mind!

I laughed, I felt giddy because in that moment, I finally accepted that unless someone can receive me exactly as I am, then I'm completely ok on my own! I'd rather be single than with someone who needs me to be 'less' or different. It took a while but I genuinely love the person I've accepted myself to be, allowing all my quirks to be visible. Yes, it makes me feel vulnerable but it mainly makes me feel honest and liberated and empowered and very, very real.

I've learnt that the right people will receive you and love you exactly as you are because you're being true to yourself and that has the magnificent ripple of giving other people permission to do the same! Like-minded people will gravitate towards you, so don't dim your light or shrink under others people's opinion and certainly don't apologise for not being everyone's cup of tea!

"Right after her birth, Eliane and I looked at each other. Her radiant, wise presence said, 'Are you here for me? Are you ready to do this?'. It awoke a decision within me to show up fully expressed, for her and for me. To be and to do what I came here to do."

And Elisabeth kept her promise to her children, using her voice as their mother, seeing their potential and walking the fine line between standing up for them and holding space for their own voices to emerge.

She also uses her voice as a mystic, entering the spiritual realms and as a composer and singer, creating healing potions!

@elisabethdecharondestgermain

Elisabeth de Charon de Saint Germain

It's OK to Invite Truth

It was barely three weeks into the new year, cozied up in our bed with coffee, when my husband shared his struggle of repressing his bisexuality. He told me how he'd been seeing another man for a couple of months behind my back and although he was deeply remorseful for having kept it a secret, he felt finally able to embrace himself for who he was.

I became very quiet. I saw an aliveness in his face as he explained that I hadn't seen for many years, his face that I so loved. He expected my rage. But I saw a light coming into my heart and into the room. Something inside me said, 'This is it my love, the moment you were waiting for. There is nothing to fear'.

He shared it all and held nothing back, even when I asked all my questions. A strange relief washed over me. The times I'd convinced myself I was wrong, it turned out my intuition was right.

I also saw my own repression, where I'd settled for being loved 'less than', I'd longed For, I saw it on his face as well. Here it was. This deeply intimate space with the truth of who we were. And all this love between us. I had longed for a fully expressed life and a love based in authenticity for as long as I can remember. Now it had arrived, it looked weird. It was hard to get my head around and surely nothing like any romcom I'd ever seen.

But damn! It sure brought me on a magical journey that opened the gate to more love and aliveness within myself than any Disney story could've given me.

Love is a power like no other. It grows with truth. When you're anxious to look at the truth of the state of your relationship, know it's okay to let the truth in, my love. The truth will return your divine, fierce and powerful feminine energy back to you.

With this activated power you can face anything and thrive, whether it is within or without your current relationship.

CALL BACK THE GODDESS

I still remember the look of delightful surprise on my first serious boyfriend's face. I was fifteen and he was five years older, when my love for him met the depths of my full feminine sensual energy. Something so powerful streamed from my lips into his that I felt, for the first time, my ancient goddess power stirring within me.

She was unashamed, fierce, loving, passionate, sexual, nurturing, playful, wise and above all, radiating a sense of sacred sensual confidence!

Between that very first stirring and right before I turned fifty, my inner goddess hid herself many times. I silenced her, it was too painful to invite her when lovers and boyfriends tried to tame or possess her. Or, even worse, during the long periods when my husband didn't desire her at all. I'd started to believe that she was a disturbing energy. I just needed to learn not to be 'so much', not to be so passionate, didn't I?

I tried to intellectualise, spiritualise and work myself away from my own sensual goddess power. But when it turned out it had all been for nothing, she fully reclaimed her space. I trusted her voice and guidance. She taught me my sacred 'yes' and my sacred 'no'. I stopped being so afraid of my shadow aspects and integrated them with love.

It was a wild ride that asked for a lot of attention, learning and the untangling of old patterns that where like poison to my system. Slowly, I opened an energetic pathway for my own self-love and my beloveds - the one who's presence can invite all of her into the space.

My most precious discovery however, is that she is me! Since inviting her back, my creative energy soared, my new romantic partner opened this sacred delightful softness within me and the platonic love between my husband and I, is now highly supportive and a source of joy.

Having access to your full expression makes so much more possible. Find the courage to remember what part of you you've hidden away. Feel into it, call your goddess back darling.

BRING LOVING INTENT INTO CHAOS

When you feel a revolution is at hand...take your leadership, plan with loving intent and then leave some space for magic. When the new reality of my marriage turned out to be more 'Pirates of the Caribbean' anarchistic than Cinderella predictable, I faced two colliding worlds. One loaded with pain and the other, holding all the opportunities and dreams I had neatly tucked away and out of sight. I so wanted to say yes to both.

I said to myself...'Here is the revolution you wanted to be in but it's not just you and him, it's the children, it's the company, it's your physical and mental health. You are smart and courageous but you're not able to do it alone. You have friends and family. Bring them in'.

I made a list of needs and wants. I looked ahead for what might come up. To tell you the truth, I felt like a General planning for wartime, except that I planned like a woman and wanted no casualties. I explained the situation to my siblings and asked them to be on standby for our children in case they needed to vent their anger or grief when the time came.

I planned like our lives depended on it. Re-creating an existing marriage is one thing, knowing yourself enough to not want to be traumatised further, is another and equally important thing. We consciously built a network of trusted people around us and asked for help.

We created this new chapter with clarity, allowed space for the raw truth of our emotions and invited our wisdom to join us. We planned for integration time, for space...revolution brings chaos.

When you bring loving intent into the chaos, you'll see a butterfly emerge from her chrysalis.

SOURCE HAS NO LIMITING BELIEF SYSTEM

An accident on a bridge had me hanging between two pieces of steel. In pain and fear, possibly about to give up, a strange relief came over me when I felt warm trickling pee running down my legs. After that, everything changed. I found myself in a fast-moving film, showing me an overview of my then eleven-year-old Self. Through a closing lens, I landed back in the same world I'd been thrown out of just a nano-second before.

This time I felt no pain, no worry and absolutely no fear. My worldview forever shifted in this moment when I saw, heard, felt and understood the interconnected deep loving and wise web of every creature, element, molecule and conscious-filled-intelligence around me. Everything was communicating with and in service of, each other.

From the singing bird, to the sunbeams on the water, all creation was sacred, loved, and valued evenly, by a Source that, without any judgement, held this fabric together.

My near-death-experience was a gift that became my North-Star, liberating me from my mother's debilitating hierarchical, transactional and black-and-white belief system, I was reconnected with my own direct lifeline with Source.

All of us are loved. If you ever doubt that your 'truth' is a bad thing, know that Source never asks you to conform to any limiting belief system. Source casts no judgement and it doesn't ask you to prove, do or earn your place in the sun. Saying 'yes' to yourself allows your unique divine design to unfold and work within you.

The day you fall in love with yourself is the day you open the door to divinely thrive.

YOU CARRY YOUR OWN MEDICINE

Medicine is not only a substance used in the treatment of a disease. The Latin etymology of the word 'medicina' speaks of 'the healing art, medicine; a remedy'. As a small girl at night, in the safe space of my own room, I used to sing out loud for hours. In this somewhat trance like state, my racing thoughts came to rest and my anxiety vanished.

These wordless songs that came out of my fantasy and rose from my body, were medicine for my soul. Singing made me feel all my emotions and transformed them into harmony. I sang my joy, as much as I sang my confusions and my pains. Where I could give no words for childhood's wounds, I sang them. Long before I became a professional singer and composer, the medicine already was there! It's there for everybody.

You don't need to be talented or become a professional artist to wake this medicine up within you. The simple act of connecting with your breath and the sound of your own voice plus your imaginative awareness, will give you access to this healing art.

Find a quiet space, in nature or in your home. Feel your body held into the love of mother earth. Imagine she asks you to share your heart with her. Feel what comes up and notice what energy it has. What element do you feel? Air? Water? Fire? Earth? Let your voice and your being merge with that element.

Trust the sacred wisdom of your voice. Share yourself and let your song be received by mother earth and your own heart. Don't analyse it, just shift from one frequency into the other. There's a point where the healing silence enters. Be still. Listen for the resonance and acknowledge how your cells are nurtured, loved and healed by the echo of your own voice.

The stillness is where the biggest healing takes place.

THE DREAM OF YOUR SOUL IS FOUND WITHIN YOUR HEART

I had such fantastic dreams as a child. I had a burning desire to become this courageous knight, in service for peace and love, always in search of cosmic wisdom and higher magic.

I longed for adventure and becoming friends with the unknown. At night my lucid dreams pulled me towards the most joyful music up into the mountains, where I sang and danced with this orchestra of celestial beings, small planets and friendly creatures, who were themselves, the instruments.

In the day, I could still hear and feel my singing voice. Like the music patterns I inwardly heard and saw, I knew the freedom of my voice. Honestly, from my teens until my mid-forties I desperately tried to dream dreams that made sense to others. But I never fully fitted into any of them. Not as a classical singer, an entrepreneur, a feminine leadership coach or as a woman.

Only after becoming fifty, amid my soul's dark night, did I stop conforming to normalcy. I surrendered to being me: I am a Mystic. Always have been. My songs and music are filled with light codes that activate sacred magic. My life, love and work look completely unconventional but I now experience a deep-rooted harmonic frequency of peace and joy within me.

Right now, you might be at a place where nothing makes sense. With the obvious dreams gone, it's time to surrender. Put your hand on your heart, breathe into it and ask your heart to bring up the dreams you brought with you to this planet.

Invite your heart to ignite the dream of your soul. Observe, acknowledge and let it be your guiding light.

ALLOW YOUR VOICE TO BE ALL THAT IT IS

"I want my voice to be as expressive, touching and free as yours", people have said to me. And I say in return, "Your voice will find its freedom and strength when you stop putting expectations upon it".

All I needed 'to do' to find my voice, was to love and allow it to be ALL that it was. I felt that if I couldn't love my voice, the way it sounded, sang or spoke, then I was cutting off my deepest soul connection. I couldn't define what my voice was capable of from that place of lack and insecurity, I was shutting down the true gift my voice wanted me to receive.

So, listen to yourself with love and interest, just observe and find the fun, the character and your uniqueness, as it is now.

Be curious. Be gentle. Have fun. You and your voice have a lifetime of exploring to do. Allow it to pull you to a place where it feels blissfully good. When I did that, something amazing happened, I met the stream of consciousness my voice was connected to and I gained a complete sense of joy and reverence.

WRITE YOUR LIFE AS YOU WANT IT

For a large part of my life and career, I'd felt driven by two forces. One, was an unconditional loving force, I sense it through the whole fabric of nature...that we are connected to Source. The other was a darker force. It felt like a pressure that constantly had me proving my worth...'If you want to enjoy the fun, you better work for it!'. It felt heavy and stressed me out. I couldn't keep up with its insatiable hunger.

My life looked like a soap opera at times, until I realised that my life was a play and I was its writer. I realised that words carry a powerful manifesting energy. I began rewriting my stories by carefully observing the energetic effects that my words had on my nervous system.

When the narrative of old sob stories made me feel yucky, I changed them by acknowledging my victorious moments too. When I wanted my dreams to come true, I'd put myself in a high vibe space and speak and write about them, as if they'd already happened. My internal system felt lighter.

Battling with inner and outer conflicts means dancing with them. My negative self-talk drastically changed towards internal kindness. This simple adjustment has had quite a miraculous effect. I use uplifting words daily and I've rewritten disempowering stories by noticing the hidden gifts they offered.

My mental and physical health had a stellar improvement, my dream house in the middle of nature with the sweet fireplace and bath, effortlessly landed in my lap and the way my romantic soulmate matched my deepest desires, when he walked into my story was actually quite miraculous.

When you're living a story that's not serving your highest good, if there's more drama than adventure, realise that you have the freedom to change it. Becoming a conscious writer of your life works best by doing it often, while using the high vibes of self-care activities like dancing, baths or finding sacred spaces in nature.

When your frequency is high, get your journal out. Find the gold hidden within the shadows. Speak and journal about those dreams you want to manifest in the present or even past tense. And mostly, speak to yourself with kindness and love.

Speak to yourself with kindness

Iona's mum lived and died with bravery, grace, and compassion. She lived her life following her adventurous heart, bravely stepping out of societal conditioning. She loved fiercely and left a legacy for her daughter.

Iona has gone on to follow in her mother's footsteps by using her voice in roles that support others. As an adviser within the Citizens Advice Bureau, for the homeless, in court appeals and as a special advocate for children, Iona has been an incredible strength to many.

Now, as a coach and healer for women, she inspires women to live with freedom, grace, and impact, just as her mother did. She wanted to be part of this movement of women in this book, supporting women and children in Bali and understanding the massive ripple effect it will have.

@iamionarussell

IONA RUSSELL

BREATHE IN SLOWLY TO HELP YOU BE PRESENT

When I'm feeling overwhelmed or stuck, I think of it these days as being disconnected from what's happening right now. I'm probably distracted, caught up in either past or future thinking.

My heart rate rises, I feel a rush of heat through my body like a pressure cooker with all the steam compounding in my head. Sometimes I get a sudden sense of prickly heat in my hands – that's my sign to bring myself back to the present.

I stop what I'm doing and breathe in slowly through my nose to fill my belly and then I breathe out through the mouth. I imagine that my breath is coming in and out of my heart.

As I feel calmer, I try to find three things that I'm grateful for. If I'm able, I like to go outside and stand barefoot on the grass while I do this. I can feel my heart rate slow, my whole body relax and a sense of peace wash over me.

In that calm state, I've noticed that I can be really creative with my writing and painting. Currently I've contributed to seven books, written a number of articles in magazines and I've painted so many pieces of art, my son wants me to sell them!

When you're present and in gratitude, I believe we open ourselves up to creativity and inspiration. Breathe in my love and breathe out slowly, everything's ok.

IT'S TIME TO LET IT GO AND FORGIVE MY DEAR

I'd been angry at my father since I was eight years old. This was the beginning of a challenging relationship with him and his authoritarian parenting style. I rebelled against it my whole life and from the age of seventeen to thirty-two, I didn't speak to him.

For much of that time, I got on with my life and he with his but I knew I needed to heal those feelings within me.

It wasn't until I started to explore less traditional therapies that I began to truly heal my mindset and internal unconscious thoughts and feelings. Energy work helped, so did past life healing, hypnosis and meditation was on my list too.

I had what I would call a return to the embodied philosophical, psychological and spiritual way of living. That brought with it, inner peace and healing...a return to a connection between my own mind, body and soul.

Recently I visited him and for the first time in my adult life, I felt a rush of love and compassion. In that moment, there was nothing to forgive, I literally felt the last remnants of anger evaporate.

A deep inner peace now envelops me. Forgiveness is the inner work of healing yourself. It's time to let it go and forgive my dear.

BE REBELLIOUS, EMBRACE YOUR INNER WILD CHILD

As a teenager I was creative with my self-expression and determined in my views. I didn't question who I was or at least I wasn't afraid to try something new, with varying degrees of 'success' I see on reflection, from my now fifty plus years. I love the girl I was and I wish she'd have known how precious she was back then.

I didn't try to fit in and was sometimes quirky and awkward, other times daring and revealing but always kind and compassionate with a zest for life. I was especially rebellious where my hair was concerned. I've had my hair every colour under the sun from a jet-black half shaved Mohican, to a blonde pixie then an orange flame of overly henna-dyed hair. It once turned green when I tried to dye it blue, I had an eighties fried perm and the nineties quiff of Rachel-esque locks.

This, is a short (pardon the pun) example of how I have been rebellious and creative. See this as your invitation to do the same. Let go of convention, embrace your inner wild child, express yourself!

CHOOSE A WAY TO MEDITATE THAT BRINGS YOU PEACE

It was midnight. I was two years into my marriage and I felt a pressing and overwhelming sense of dread and sadness. I sat bolt upright in bed and through tears, said to my then husband "I can't do this anymore".

I thought we had to change our location, I thought my husband needed to change or my son had to change. I thought something, maybe everyone (outside of me) had to change!

I went looking for all the answers...I took courses, connected with wisdom seekers, gathered books on everything from spirituality to neuroscience and then I stumbled into a non-denominational meditation group.

I grew up with Buddhist parents. Meditation was part of my early years, until I rebelled and sought external means of gratification. I call these the wilderness years.

I didn't have a 'normal' upbringing, it was free-range and spiritually led, so meditation was like coming home to me, to my own heart and wholeness.

Daily meditation meant I finally found what I'd been looking for, like some big cosmic joke, it was ME. Somewhere over the previous four decades, I'd lost 'me'.

I found a sense of inner peace. All I needed to do was accept myself and be ok with me as I am. Like a pool of water - you keep throwing rocks in, hoping they'll settle, thinking one more rock will help but it's when you stop, that the ripples gradually slow, calm and settle...meditation was that for me. Something else might bring you peace, we don't all have to sit cross legged on the floor for hours but find peace for ten minutes twice a day.

Begin breathing, focusing on the breath with music or silence. Let it be easy. Do what you need in the moment...and the last secret...when you don't think you have time to meditate, that's when you need it most!

EXPRESS YOURSELF

Years ago, I started down the path of an eating disorder based on an innocent comment by a friend. She said she'd rather be fat and happy like me, than thin and miserable. I'd never thought about my weight until then. I was thirteen. There were other issues at play but that's the moment I remember first viewing myself as fat. In fact, I was beautiful.

I didn't think I looked like others did, I felt I wasn't good enough. I controlled my eating which lasted two weeks before I was so hungry, I went to the other extreme of binge eating and purging...I thought I'd found the holy grail!

As I got thinner, I got so many compliments on my looks, that it just reinforced I wasn't acceptable as I was. Like a spiral, it continued. Over the years, it tapered off but was always a thing I did to 'feel better'. It plagued me into adulthood like a dirty little secret and a comforting security blanket, just there, like weaning off a drug, sometimes I just needed one last fix. Recovery wasn't a quick fix, it was gradual.

The more confident I became, the more I accepted myself. I nurtured my inner child, to look at myself and see that beautiful thirteen-year-old.

I no longer stuff my feelings down or judge myself. It took time and it took doing the inner work of self-love to get where I am now. I love food, it nourishes me, feeds me and keeps my body healthy. I love cooking for others, an expression of love I channelled, to share.

My love, it's time to move from suppression to the expression of your divine magic – express your true self.

LISTEN TO THE WHISPERS FOR ADVENTURE AND CURIOSITY!

I have lived with a wild hearted curiosity for adventure. While some called me fool hearted, others envied my escapades. I leapt at opportunities as they appeared, which always led to unexpected connections and possibilities. Every lesson a learning experience, as I've travelled wearing many work hats along the way; backpacking alone through Europe at twenty, nannying in Hawaii at twenty-one, driving a campervan across Australia by twenty-seven and getting my motorbike licence in Scotland at thirty-one.

Each adventure led to the next and I absolutely could not have foretold or predicted where my life path would take me. I became a child advocate in Texas in my early forties and flew microlight planes through the Himalayas at forty-seven with my thirteen-year-old. I published my first book aged forty-nine and now at fifty-two, I've contributed to seven books with my second solo one on the way.

The point is, we're never too young or too old for wild hearted adventures in life. If whispers are calling you, go...maybe I'll see you there on the horizon!

PLACE YOUR HAND ON YOUR HEART

A tree grows its roots deep into the earth. It's balanced by the equal reach of its branches and without those strong deep roots, it's easily uprooted and knocked off balance in turbulent times. A tree that is rigid and unwavering, will snap and crack in the changing winds of time.

When I become unsteady emotionally or physically, part of what I've learnt that it's because I've lost connection to myself and mother earth. I was taught that the thinking mind is the aspect of us we should value above all else, so I became overly head-led, trapped by analytical thinking. I felt like a prisoner to worry and anxiety, it caused me to be unsteady and doubt myself so many times.

To find the harmony and the equilibrium again, I got into a practice of placing my hand on my heart. For me, this is the secret to being like the deeply rooted tree, it gives me the ability to sway and move with the changing seasons of my life.

You are of mother earth, your heart is the portal to connection between you and her. When we connect to her through our hearts, there are no right or wrong answers, from this place of calm, you can make grounded decisions.

This is a practise. Life is a practise, it's all ok.

YOU ARE ABUNDANT

I didn't always think this way. In doing my own inner work and working on my self-worth, I realised I didn't value myself and I didn't feel abundant. I felt lack. I wanted others to approve my worth by fitting in...drinking to excess, putting on a mask, being promiscuous etc.

I thought abundance was all about money and I had conflicting ideas around that. I felt ashamed if I had money when others didn't, I self-sabotaged and was overly generous (maybe again for approval and acceptance). I perceived those who didn't have money as being happier, more fun-loving and community based, so I wanted to live on the local council estate rather than on a farm in the mountains. All those kids outside playing together, I felt liberated being with them.

I know now that abundance is about ALL areas of life...health, wealth, relationships, connection, contribution to the world, impact, family. Abundance is less about the limited material world and more about the infinite world within us.

The paradigm-shifting truth is, we are all naturally abundant, we always have access to the bountiful and ever-generous spiritual domain and we can tap into the abundance of life and the universe at any time.

In abundance, you see only plenty. Your heart is full. Your soul expands. You're rooted, in flow, soaring and alight, all at once.

There's a natural confidence that comes when you live in certainty of your own inner and outer wealth. The right people and opportunities come when you walk your prosperous path and it starts with being grateful. Find the seeds of the gratitude. Life can be hard, so look for the silver lining.

Sue's reaction was immediate and heartfelt upon receiving the invitation to contribute to this book. "I felt the emotion, excitement and importance of sharing as soon as I read the invitation to write [this book], I listened to my hearts call", she recounted and we couldn't be happier that she did!

Her parents played a pivotal role during her early years, guiding her in finding her voice. Over time, through experiences as diverse as being a sailing crew member, leading in the corporate world, facing life's emergencies and directing retreats, she has honed her voice - understanding its softness as well as its assertiveness.

She hopes that you, dear reader, will find within her words a source of strength, a companion and a space to pause, reflect and listen to your own heart.

@tranquilitytimesue

SUE ROYLE

START THE DAY WITH SPACE FOR YOU

Twenty years ago, I used to leave my yoga session before the end. I thought I'd fulfilled my physical needs, I didn't think the lying down bit at the end was necessary. I now know it's THE most valuable part for me. It resets my nervous system, I sleep better and I'm happier.

I need that space. When I don't have it, I'm impatient, I lack focus and creativity...my spark like a weak flame.

So I make that space for myself at the start of my day and if my mind tells me I don't have time, I need it even more.

Some mornings I walk barefoot in the garden. I take deep breaths. If I'm tired, I sit with my hands wrapped around a hot mug and savour those first few sips of comfort and nurturing warmth while I watch the birds. Sometimes I listen to music. But whatever I do, I set up my day.

It dictates how my day unfolds. I'm nicer to myself, kinder to everyone else and I meet challenges with more patience.

Just one moment of morning magic. can miraculously make your day more easeful and peaceful.

Even if you have a hectic schedule, just a few moments placing your hand on your belly, feeling the rise and fall of the breath, is a beautiful way of just being.

MEDITATE, HOLD SPACE FOR YOURSELF

I cannot express enough, the relevance and reward I have found in meditating. When I take time to sit and embrace stillness, especially when outside, with Mother Nature, I feel she reveals so many secrets, almost as if rewarding my patience for the space I hold for myself.

Birds come a little closer as if they sensed the safety of my stillness and stayed a little longer. The wind blows more gently and the warmth of the sun feels so welcome...as if it relaxes the deepest parts of my soul.

As I slowly open my eyes, when I awaken from meditation, I feel humbled and delighted to share these few moments of magic. I am once again, back in rhythm, with richness of life in the moment.

It's my answer to finding balance in life...simply meditate in a way that works for you and the space will embrace you and allow you to be.

DO THINGS THAT TAKE YOU OUTSIDE YOUR COMFORT ZONE

Each time a new opportunity arises, it's the same. First, I feel excited and my eyes shine for adventure, then logic kicks in. A sensible and protective line of questioning starts...I feel like it's a built-in survival reaction to keep me safe but I also feel that if I'd have listened to that protective part of me, I'd never have embraced the adventures I have...and they were great!

I would have worried about what might happen if something went wrong in that sailing race, I admit to thinking about what would happen if I got bitten by a mosquito in India, I also wondered what would happen if I had a panic attack on the paddle board in the middle of the ocean!

But I did them anyway. Let me tell you, I expanded WAY beyond my comfort zone. I would have been quite happy, safe and content on my sofa at home but I wouldn't have grown in the same way, I wouldn't have encountered the same emotions or seen the things I have. I can say, hand on heart, they absolutely changed my life!

Those things ignited passion in me, they ignited action and motivation. I've been inspired and had my soul humbled by the beauty of other cultures and how content they are to simply be alive.

I've lived where smiling to strangers and placing a hand on your heart as a greeting is the norm! It's had such a profound effect on me! I've spent times out at sea, with a crew not knowing if we'd make it back safely...just praying that we did and I mean quite literally praying!

In my experience, we have to listen to our soul, to our heart not our head. Step outside the circle of the known, straight into the unknown...the best gift of all may just be waiting there for you, undiscovered.

TRUST IN THE TIMING

I always had leapt from one relationship to another, spending little time on my own but this was marriage! You're supposed to stay married! What would people say? I had failed...it was so sad but we both knew it wasn't right. We parted still caring for one another. Every day for six months I cried on the train to work. I felt empty and lost. But once I got to London, it was almost like I'd stepped into another world and I would pull myself together, put some makeup on, get my heels on and walk to the office.

I worked hard and partied hard but it was when I arrived home at night to an empty, cold, dark house, it always really hit me. I wondered what I had done, questioned if I'd done the right thing.

I found myself living on big lunches at work and toast for tea, sometimes a pack of chocolate digestives and a film. I stayed up late not wanting to go to bed alone but slowly of course, I started to relax. The tears gradually stopped and my new life began.

I learned to love this time with myself. I found a new routine. Adventures opened up and I found myself travelling, doing things I would never have done before. I grew and gained confidence, girlfriends gathered and gave support. The new chapter began.

I had to go through this emotional turmoil, to truly see myself, to spend time with Susan and learn that life with me was fun. I learned that I was good company, that I could survive on my own. If you find yourself in this situation, you have the answers within, just listen and trust.

Your true friends will stay close, you'll be amazed at your own courage and at the wisdom and resourcefulness that will reach you in your moments of despair. You will be ignited once again and your next adventure will unfold.

Don't hide who you really are

It wasn't until I started school and began telling stories of what I'd done in the holidays that I realised, I liked different things to my friends. I loved being out in nature, staying out as late as I could and when I had to come in, I'd write stories of the adventures my cat and I had had to other magical worlds.

I was interested in crystals and moon cycles and pebbles but as I got older, I hid it all, so I could fit in. I got engrossed in a fast-paced corporate life and much later, at a life cross roads, I went for a card reading with a medium.

"You know you don't really need to come to me, don't you" she said, "You could do this yourself", I thought she was joking. But then I realised, my interests as a child were the clue that everything I needed was within, just hidden. I started going to mediumship circles, growing more confident and aware of what was available within me, that had always been available within me.

Initially, I still hid, I told my partner I was going out with friends when in fact, I was giving readings and learning about Angel cards and Mediumship...most importantly...I was learning how to be me!

Eventually I told him and he wasn't in the least bit bothered. So, don't hide away. Learn who you are. I'm so pleased this work is now part of my business.

I share my stories and teachings and I've found that the right people arrive if you're truly yourself and able to trust your own gifts!

JUMP SHIP TO BECOME SELF EMPLOYED

Moving into my new house brought tears of joy! It also brought a bigger mortgage! That was ok though, I worked in London, I had it covered. I'd just get up earlier to catch the train, it'd be fine. I'd have done anything for the walks and spectacular sunrises and moonsets that my new house had!

In reality, I was up earlier than the sun and too exhausted to even notice the moon. At that time, I was still very 'in my head' so, I'm still surprised by what came next. I resigned! I wanted to see the magic of the elements and the skies reflecting in the water, I wanted to be here in that house every morning, every day!

So I did it. I handed my notice in and just like that I was free. My husband thought I was mad, he said it was an 'airy fairy' idea but I knew.

Morning sunrises and dog walks gave me freedom and yes there was fear, I'd left a secure job with a good salary...but I'd been offered a job two days a week, enough to cover my bills and it gave me belief and confidence!

The support from business owners in my new location was abundant, I'm ever grateful to them and I now run two businesses! So, trust your heart, believe in yourself, we all have it within us and it's just waiting to be awoken!

FIND YOUR SOUL SOUND

I believe we should all have at least one thing we can get lost in. One thing that feeds our soul, fills our heart with joy, keeps us grounded and lights us up.

I believe that when we find that one thing, then we can tap into it at any time – it brings us back to who we are. I've heard that we all have our own 'soul sound' when we're breathed into existence. For me, it's singing. I like doing many things but when I sing...it lights me up FULLY!

It transforms my mood, my mind can't wander anywhere, I'm focused. When I sing, I am completely and fully in that note. I feel so much joy, so much pleasure, I'm so uplifted, sometimes I can't believe the sounds that are coming from deep within me. I am truly in-the-moment when I sing. Find your own soul sound, the one thing that brings you back to who you truly are.

MANIFESTATION IS REAL, INVITE IN ABUNDANCE

I'm still not sure whether it was the jet lag, the Indian magic or having recently skimmed the book 'The Secret' but suddenly, I remembered...apparently, all I had to do was believe.

I grabbed my pen and paper before I changed my mind and started writing, no holds barred. I listed everything I wished for and this time, I believed!

The dream house, the river, the land, the fishing rights, the moorings, the chickens, the spacious light buildings, the wildlife and the woodland walks! I didn't just think with my head, I allowed my heart to write. I signed it, sealed it in an envelope, putting a date for it to arrive by on the back.

I placed it where I could see it every day. A few months later, our house sold and we found the house...with everything I'd listed!

Three other buyers popped in blind bids but I knew it was ours! I didn't even need to see the inside, the energy was perfect and just standing outside it made my eyes fill up with tears.

I cut the picture of it out from the brochure and stuck it on my desk at work. I changed the colour of the garage doors to the colour I would paint them when it was ours and it was! The date on envelope was 1st August 2013 and we moved in on 2nd!

Manifestation is real, invite in abundance!

Carol's grandmother was a strong no-nonsense woman: forthright, independent and never shy of speaking her truth.

Observing her grandmother's assertiveness in her formative years left a deep imprint on Carol; she recalls standing up for herself from the earliest memories of her childhood.

Her journey from adolescence to adulthood, from exploration during her travels to being a wife, a mother, a friend and eventually a widow, has been marked by the confident use of her voice.

She wishes every woman who reads this book peace, trust and a knowing that she is exactly where she is meant to be.

@lifestyle_fitness_consultants

CAROL O'CONNOR

LONELINESS, UNDERSTAND AND APPRECIATE YOURSELF

I think feeling alone and being alone are two very different animals. Until I was fifty, I'd always lived with people...family, friends, husband, kids and...I still had feelings of loneliness sometimes.

It was only when I was totally on my own, when my husband died and both my sons went off to university that I really sat with 'loneliness' and got curious about it.

When I accepted my loneliness, I discovered something powerful and freeing on the other side. I discovered that certain journeys cannot be taken unless we're willing to face loneliness, yet so many of us are afraid to do that. For inner growth, I now believe, it's a 'must-do', to do that work.

That said, to appreciate time alone, most of us need to feel we have a choice, that friends or family are close by when needed. If not, time alone can be miserable.

Place your hand on your heart, close your eyes, take a deep breath in, it calms the mind. Make peace with yourself and all that has come before. Take another deep breath in, decide if you need to cry alone or with someone else. It's all healing.

THE PEACE AND FREEDOM YOU DESIRE IS ALREADY WITHIN YOU

I've worked harder than I should have in my life. I've travelled to many countries, put other people's needs before my own, I've been so generous with my time and my energy. In short, I spent many years trying to please everyone. To the detriment of my own health.

None of that gave me the peace and freedom I sought. That only came when I sat alone with myself and with the uncomfortable and sometimes scary feelings of being on my own, of not being understood and of not quite fitting in.

I breathed into those feelings. I let them sit with me, I let them move through me. Sometimes, they're still there but I got comfortable with them and now when they visit, I treat them like old friends! The sensations they created are so familiar, bloody uncomfortable but familiar nevertheless. I don't try and ignore them.

PAUSE, LOOK UP and BREATHE my love. You are the master of your own internal universe, your thoughts and feelings.

The peace and freedom you desire and crave is already within you.

LISTENING TO YOUR GUT

It's never wrong. Time and time again my gut instinct has shown me so. It's always been there bubbling away in the back ground, I just had to listen to it.

The general noise from my life, my friends and family pressures, meant I spent a lot of time disconnected from it. The more I pause to connect back to my innate wisdom/inner voice though, the more I hear. I do this in many ways. Mediation, journalling, focusing on my breath, exercising and being outdoors all help me.

When I pause and become physically still, I am able to hear and feel. There's not always a big light bulb moment (although they are great when they happen) but I can definitely feel the benefit.

Be prepared, listening to your gut and acting on it, can upset those around you. I've fallen out with enough of them to know it well but while others think they know what's best for us, they really don't.

I'm a logical person, so I use logic with my instinct. I research, it's like a comfort blanket around my gut! But by following it, I left my hometown in my twenties, packed in a promising career and moved overseas with nothing but a deep knowing that there was more for me in life!

I've taken jobs, changed careers, called off an engagement, chosen lovers and partners, bought houses...all... while others thought I was crazy. I even feel that listening to my gut, saved my life from potentially dying of cancer. It's always with you, just quieten the external noise to hear it, then over prepare and go with the flow!

BEING PRESENT – THE GIFT THAT KEEPS ON GIVING

Many years ago, I had one of those BOOM moments when my youngest son, who was about nine years old, said "But mum the present is the gift!". 'Wow' I thought, so simple but so profound. We weren't doing anything special; I think he was being a typical child lost in thought and I was trying to tell him something.

It got me thinking. I'd spent much of my adult life worrying about what I had or hadn't done, striving for something bigger or better...the job, the handbag, the boyfriend, the lover, the experience, the emotion...always striving, never satisfied.

I'd either be stressing about the past (which is a total waste of time as we all know it cannot be changed) or worrying about the future, for which I don't believe we have much control over.

In doing that, I realised that I really don't remember many of my achievements. I mean…I can list them sure but I don't remember how they felt emotionally!

Part of me feels I missed all the joyous emotions back when they happened. I often struggle to recall the memories. I try now not to live with regrets but it's definitely the small things I never took time to appreciate or absorb that saddens me.

I have found a fabulous way to help me connect and be present though. I connect to my five senses…sound, smell, sight, taste and touch. They help to slow me down and ground me enough to live for the moment. I've never forgotten my sons words and I live now, seeing the present moment as a gift.

FLOW THROUGH GRIEF

I spent too many years suppressing grief. I can see now that my survival depended on it but I realised at some point, that if I continued to suppress it, it might never heal.

As a doer, a high achiever and a perfectionist, I'd never noticed I wasn't processing it. Grief for me started at a very young age, from the childhood I thought I should've had, to becoming a widow in my forties but it wasn't until I was diagnosed with cancer and was forced to slow down, that I found out I had indeed been suppressing it and that I needed to put it to rest. That meant there was an awful lot of it to work through!

Messy and painful, there didn't seem to be any right or wrong way, any 'perfect time' or space, to do that deep work. It was a journey of self-discovery. I worked with a counsellor and a few close friends who supported me without trying to fix me. I also had to let go of how far along the path I thought I 'should' be! And while it's still a work in progress, it's not something to be fixed. I believe grief becomes a part of the tapestry of life. It hasn't shrunk but over time, my world has got bigger around it.

I still have days where I pick myself off the floor and dust myself down, to crack back on with living in this beautiful, wonderful incredible life we have been given. Life is full of loss and grief; it's simply a natural part of the healing process and as the saying goes 'what doesn't kill you makes you stronger'. You will flow through it my love.

FOCUS ON BEING GRATEFUL FOR SMALL THINGS

When I practice gratitude, I notice that there's a lot more to be grateful for. In my younger years, I didn't really allow myself to be grateful for all the things I did or achieved, I always thought I should be doing more.

I definitely came from a place of never feeling like I was enough. I tried though, I kept a gratitude diary but even though I was writing things in it, I still felt there was something deep inside me that was never truly satisfied. Fast forward a few years and a string of life-changing traumatic events, gratitude has now become a very strong and real trait in my very existence, my mood and emotions.

When I live from a place of gratitude, I find I have more to give. When I no longer focus on what I lack, gratitude strengthens relationships with my family and friends and I've seen that I can't be angry, scared or lonely and grateful at the same time.

In cultivating a sense of gratitude, I've actually got rid of most of my negative feelings and they've been replaced with an inner peace and joy. Appreciating the little things in life means I focus my attention on what nurtures and sustains me. All that truly matters in the end, is that you loved. Know, dear one, that the best is yet to come.

IT'S OK TO SAY HOW YOU FEEL

I feel that feelings of not being loved, not being enough or not being heard, tend to develop from our childhood, if we haven't been supported, encouraged or listened to.

I was loved in some ways. I was fed and watered and I had a roof over my head but for me, it didn't seem the kind of love that nurtured my soul. Consequently, I've led a life of never feeling enough, of striving for perfection and never being satisfied. I thought the more I did, achieved or pleased others, the more I'd 'be'. If this is you STOP. It might get you noticed, you'll likely achieve great things but it won't fill you up emotionally.

You see, I wasn't aligned with my soul. I had many warning signs that I took no notice of but, eventually my wake-up call came in the form of a rare salary gland cancer tumour that grew in my lung.

Traditional Chinese medicine says we store grief in our lungs. This diagnosis showed me that by swallowing, not sharing/voicing my truth, not honouring my true feelings or emotions, not speaking up about what I really needed or wanted emotionally, can cause disease.

So, be true to yourself. Pause, check in with yourself, check in with your heart. You don't have to please anyone else or try to fit in. Speak your truth, voice what you feel and don't store your emotions, it's ok to say how you feel, then get up, get out, dress up and show up for life!

CURVE BALLS CAN BE A GIFT

Life has thrown me a few curveballs...as it does us all. Mine started from a young age. My parents divorced and I went through traumatic mental and physical abuse.

More recently, I lost my husband to cancer before I was fifty, becoming a solo parent, then lost my mother also to cancer soon after. To top it off, I got diagnosed with a rare cancer and had to have a part of my body removed!

It's been bloody tough. I've been to some very dark places and back again but I still smile, I still rise and I still feel totally blessed to see the sunrise every day. That's the thing about curveballs; they come from every angle and at any time. The curveballs aren't the problem though, it's how we react to them that determines our fate. After so many, I now try to be curious about them and respond with gratitude that I am at least here to deal with it!

Some curveballs are needed I think, in order to make space for bigger and better things. What if, our journeys are always leading to something better, more amazing and more incredible?

Look up my love. Appreciate the small things and the moments of joy that co-exist within the curve balls. See the curve balls as a gift. Life isn't tied up with a bow but it's still a gift! Feel and notice the contrasting feelings and emotions all at once, co-existing alongside each other.

Everything's ok my love.

Lisa's spirit guides have urged her to speak up and speak out when she needs to. And she has.

She felt she had so much to share in writing her chapter. A mum to two boys, a doula, a midwife and an artist, she is not new to birthing new creations and new life.

May her words inspire you to birth your own creations, to give a voice to your feelings and needs. May you know your worth and understand your divine power as a woman through her words.

@sivopriya

LISA HARRIS

ANCESTRAL PATTERNS ARE REAL BUT YOU CAN LET THEM GO

She never felt loved. He was a perfectionist. Through his lens though, she was perfect. But life wasn't perfect. They'd been conditioned, like we all have and we grow up listening to their words, believing the fuckery of it all, feeling silent, unworthy, misplaced. Love with conditions.

Moving through life, unconsciously repeating the same patterns carried in my DNA. Winning and losing. Questioning, understanding, forgiving.

They were just repeating what they'd been subjected to, trying to fit in and be like everybody else. Being shown how fuckery can look wearing a different outfit. Still seeking approval.

I just wanted to be loved unconditionally and you know what? I was. The problem was, I didn't love myself unconditionally, so through my life I've based being loved, on being perfect.

All those heartaches and let downs. All those times at school when I had no-one to hang out with. I kept myself quiet and shy because I'd think 'Who's interested in me?', so rather than face the rejection of not being good enough, funny enough, cool enough, interesting enough, I just buried all these feelings.

I acknowledged feeling the pain of the seven-year-old and fourteen-year-old girl, I shed the limiting beliefs, feeling compassion for their mistakes, for myself. I broke the chains of ancestral patterns. I speak to the young child regularly, acknowledging the deeper layers of trauma and finding the medicine within. Finding new strength to stand in my truth and integrate her. We cry together to release the pain. Sometimes I have no idea what we're crying about but there's no need to attach a story. It feels good.

I love you. I'm sorry. Please forgive me. Thank you. (Ho'oponopono prayer)

BE FINANCIALLY INDEPENDENT, ALWAYS

My fiancé and I were living in Brighton, we both had good jobs, a nice flat and a good social life. Upon his return from a business trip to Johannesburg, he told me he'd been offered a job there. I could have a house with a swimming pool and a maid, if I wanted. He explained I wouldn't be able to work, as I would be accompanying him as his spouse on his work permit but he'd be getting a good salary so I didn't have to worry.

I jumped at the opportunity. It was hell. I was used to having my own bank account and buying anything I wanted (usually shoes!) but to then have to ask for money to put fuel in my car or go food shopping was beyond uncomfortable.

He controlled everything. We didn't even have a joint bank account. It was around that time I met a wonderful reflexologist and I was amazed at the results. My grandmother had just given me £1000 and two months later I enrolled at a school for reflexology. That evening, I said to myself 'this is your ticket out of here Lisa', and it was.

Always, always have your own income stream and bank account, be financially independent, it's worth it.

DON'T IGNORE YOUR INTUITION AND THOSE RED FLAGS

I met my second husband online! This time was different. I really loved him. He was attractive, generous, in my age bracket and most importantly, he got on well with my sons.

I'd deliberately selected someone with children so they would understand the trials and tribulations of parenting. However, there was a red flag I chose to completely disregard on our first date, he hadn't seen his own children in fifteen years!

He could easily have been sitting there with a red flashing cone on his head and I'd have ignored it and carried on sipping my cappuccino.

One year later we married and I honestly believed I would be with him for the rest of my life. The following two years broke me though...sulky behaviour, door slamming; I felt criticised for my parenting skills and felt abused. I had a highly stressful job and my son started getting into trouble.

I broke. Our final holiday was spent bickering and having make-up sex. The rose-coloured glasses smashed when he referred to my children as 'baggage'.

Heartbroken but suddenly seeing with new lenses, I realised, this wasn't about the men in my life, it was about me and I needed to stop repeating the same pattern.

More recently, I lost my husband to cancer before I was fifty, becoming a solo parent, then lost my mother also to cancer soon after. To top it off, I got diagnosed with a rare cancer and had to have a part of my body removed!

It's been bloody tough. I've been to some very dark places and back again but I still smile, I still rise and I still feel totally blessed to see the sunrise every day. That's the thing about curveballs; they come from every angle and at any time. The curveballs aren't the problem though, it's how we react to them that determines our fate. After so many, I now try to be curious about them and respond with gratitude that I am at least here to deal with it!

Some curveballs are needed I think, in order to make space for bigger and better things. What if, our journeys are always leading to something better, more amazing and more incredible?

Look up my love. Appreciate the small things and the moments of joy that co-exist within the curve balls. See the curve balls as a gift. Life isn't tied up with a bow but it's still a gift! Feel and notice the contrasting feelings and emotions all at once, co-existing alongside each other.

Everything's ok my love.

IT'S REALLY IMPORTANT TO GROW, EVOLVE AND CHANGE

Often, when we're young, we have no idea what we want to do 'when we grow up' and even once we are grown up, we're still left wondering what our purpose is.

I knew I was a quiet girl, often 'daydreaming' I only really enjoyed art, I thought I was going to be a hairdresser. At school, I was defined by my teachers as shy and lacking in confidence. My parent's 'worried about me' and said I was very quiet and timid. I disliked school and scraped through with minimal qualifications.

Contrary to the labels I was given, I went on an 18-30's holiday to Ibiza, alone, at eighteen and two years later, became a flight attendant with Virgin Atlantic. My life 'took off' from that moment. We aren't the people we're labelled when we're young. And if I'd chosen to believe that definition of myself, it may have become the self-fulfilling prophecy.

Even if you find yourself not knowing what you want in life, knowing what you don't want is enough. You don't have to mirror someone else's life. Dream big. Know that others don't define you and that their perception of you is not your truth; it's theirs. You are always growing and evolving, choose your own label and let them change over time.

LOVE YOURSELF MORE

I always had regular size breasts, an ample 34C. When I met my first husband, I'd lost a lot of weight and my breasts lost their 'perkiness'. It didn't bother me too much until he passed a comment one day.

I booked an appointment to see a surgeon. I wanted them lifted but the surgeon advised having an implant instead as it would involve less scarring. I ended up with huge boobs facing south! Over the next twenty-three years, I had implants put in, implants removed, lifts, implants in again, implants changed. I really believed I was unlovable without having aesthetically pleasing breasts.

Following the break-up from my second husband, I went on my first plant medicine healing retreat, which was a life changing experience.

Over the course of three nights, I received inner guidance that I needed to remove my implants. At the time, I thought I was imagining things or it was something I should do for health reasons. I remember sitting on the toilet, saying out loud "I don't know how or why you want me to do this but I will do it".

Three months later, I had my final surgery to have them removed. It was only then that I understood this was about self-love and acceptance.

Apart from spending a mortgage on surgery, I wish that I'd seen how we are created whole, complete and perfect as we are. That was my lesson and I'm grateful to arrive at that stage now where I feel so complete and accepting of myself.

And the one other thing I've learnt, is that men really don't care about the size or shape of your breasts, they're just grateful to be in the presence of a naked woman!

MANIFEST WITH GRATITUDE

I wasn't even aware what manifestation was but there I was at the Hilton Hotel Gatwick airport in 1991, attending my second interview. We had to try on the red uniform, my hair styled into a French plait and red lipstick applied. Walking down the walkway, I stared at the Boeing 747s lined up outside. I looked in the bathroom mirror and said to myself loudly "You're going to be on one of them". That's when my life started.

I've reinvented myself so many times, my friend says I could have my own Wikipedia page! Manifesting is easy. We do it all day long. The secret is to manifest what we actually want. We manifest things we don't want by speaking them. Words are spells! Whatever you believe, will be.

A famous quote by Henry Ford says "Whether you think you can or you can't, you're right". However, repeating something alone will not necessarily manifest.

You need to feel it, be it, live it...like it's already happened. The feeling should be excitement and trust it will happen, without any expectations how it will happen. Relinquish control.

One practice I adopted years ago, was one of giving gratitude for what I already have and what I want. I connect to my heart and speak as though it's already happened. By the nature of universal law, you receive more of the same.

I often start my day offering gratitude with a cup of cacao, always giving thanks for this magical human experience, as well as greeting the sun. I thank the birds for singing and the rain for cleansing. I thank my ancestors who have walked before me and the lessons my children bring. Thank you for all that is.

WHAT DOES FREEDOM LOOK LIKE TO YOU?

Freedom is a state of being, a feeling within which is mirrored externally. For me to experience freedom, I had to unbecome the person everyone knew; midwife, mother, partner, daughter. Instead, I birthed the artist and the creator, I started practicing transcendental meditation, I gave up the rental on my home, donated my belongings and travelled to Peru.

I lived in the Amazon rain forest with a Shipibo family for two months, living in basic conditions where electric and water were not always available. I lived appreciating waking up to beautiful sunrises and the sounds of the jungle. India too welcomed me with open arms, my soul connected and my spirit had never felt so free.

I healed my voice through devotional songs and playing harmonium (kirtan). Most recently, I travelled to Mexico with my sixteen-year-old 'unschooled' son and ran out of money...my bank balance was £2.22! I laughed loudly and said "Wow, angelic number!". I won't lie, I panicked but my trust developed into knowing that everything was unfolding for my highest good.

I was still waking up to mountains, practising Spanish with the locals. I had everything I needed in those moments and I wouldn't have traded that for a highly paid job, suburban bliss and an annual holiday!

I stopped controlling, learning to see perfection within imperfection. I saw rejection as redirection to something far greater than I could imagine and recognised stillness wasn't stagnation. I stopped looking outside for happiness, I rested, ebbed and flowed, trusted.

Don't sacrifice your freedom or sell your soul by staying in an unfulfilling job or relationship for an easy life. Be true with yourself, be true with your word and fly free.

YOU DON'T HAVE TO STAY SO LONG

It was 1996, in Brighton. My friend introduced me to the most charismatic, entertaining man. Within a few hours though, I saw him and declared him a 'dickhead' to my friend.

He spent two months making a beeline for me, the best restaurants, home-cooked gourmet meals, making Jamie Oliver look like an amateur! Despite knowing his two-timing cheating tendencies, four years later we married.

On my wedding day, I walked beside my father, thinking 'You don't love him. This is a mistake!' but it took twelve agonising years with this womanising, egomaniac, relocating to the other side of the world with him before I left. I used to spend hours and days fantasising and planning various exit strategies but could never find the courage. The day finally came when he threatened me with divorce if I went away with my friends for the weekend. I couldn't get in my car quick enough!

I jumped in my Audi with a few bottles of vodka and an overnight bag and off I went! My definitive 'Thelma and Louise' moment!

I have no regrets. I wouldn't be the woman I am today without that experience and yet...twelve years is a long time to suffer a bad relationship. You don't have to stay so long.

I wouldn't be the woman I am today
without that experience

Tara has been surrounded by incredible women who have given her the courage, confidence and conviction to use her voice. She's had to draw on that strength to speak up and be heard throughout her career.

Doing the right thing for her staff meant challenging herself to speak up in boardrooms and in public. Her best working days were those when her voice was fuelled by intuition, fact and data.

However, her internal words have always been and remain her clearest and strongest voice. "My voice became clearer and stronger," she said, as her capacity to listen grew and she found her true path. "This is the voice that brings me the most joy and happiness"

@tara_paonessa

TARA PAONESSA

IT'S SAFE TO PUT DOWN THE ROLES THAT NO LONGER SERVE YOU

"I have responsibility for my life, you have responsibility for yours"

I had a breakdown in my late thirties. My recovery depended on a residential stay in a mental health clinic. What put me in the clinic was three decades of untreated clinical depression which led to me feeling unable to manage my earth walk, literally.

The clinical depression came about by childhood trauma and as a side effect, co-dependency played out quite strongly. I learned how to play the rescuer. I took little responsibility for my own mental health and wasn't aware of my negative patterns and beliefs.

Six months after discharge, I received a curious invitation. An acquaintance of mine was travelling to Kenya, to stay with a Maasai Tribe he knew. He asked if I wanted to go. A trip into the unknown absolutely terrified me and yet, I said yes.

The universe gave me a gift on this trip, in the form of a Maasai tradition. The ritual is this. At the birth of a child, when the midwife cuts the umbilical cord she says: "I have responsibility for my life and now you have responsibility for yours".

My love, it is safe to put down roles that no longer serve you. Go gently, with love, set your burdens free, put your boundaries in place and take responsibility for only that which is yours. You've got this.

YOU ARE EXACTLY WHERE YOU'RE MEANT TO BE RIGHT NOW

By my late forties, I'd moved house twenty-two times. I'd had a senior corporate career and had run eight of my own businesses. I'd been married more than once, travelled the world, experienced life-changing events and never seemed to settle.

I was never content, constantly driven to find the next thing. Growing up with two alcoholic parents wasn't easy, nor is being a highly sensitive person in a conflicted world.

I always took my inner work seriously, owning my stuff but, deep inside, there was discombobulation which felt like I wasn't in alignment with my higher purpose.

One day, when I'd just sold and moved on from yet another business, a dear friend asked "I don't suppose you've considered that you might have ADHD?". What??? My world fell out from under my feet and I on-the-spot dismissed her. It was too much to take in. To think I might have neurodiversity and that's why I'd been struggling?

She was right. I had a neurotypical expectation of life, yet I am neurodiverse! I completely missed it and was just to used to friends and family saying "Well it's just Tara, always moving on!".

My love, if you're feeling out of alignment or discombobulated, be open to the idea that there might be things you don't know about yourself yet. Be gentle, be kind and trust that they'll reveal themselves when the time is right. Getting to know ourselves is a precious process to be embraced, as we find our flow at each new stage.

You are exactly where you're meant to be right now. My love, trust that everything is revealed to you and comes to you in the perfect time sequence. And breathe.

ASK YOURSELF GOOD QUESTIONS

At the time of writing this chapter, I'm with my dad. He's in a nursing home, in the late stages of Alzheimer's. Sitting by his bedside, holding his hand, is the greatest gift that has been bestowed on me.

Mum passed away unexpectedly a few years ago. It was a shock and whilst we had spoken that morning and ended the conversation with "I love you", there was so much left unsaid. My internal grieving process after she passed was fairly messy. Six months after she died, my family and I relocated. I felt the sadness of leaving our home and friends, added to the grief of losing mum, I became very ill.

Because of two loving and unconventional parents, my life so far has been extraordinary. Yes, there have been some serious difficulties to overcome but they have taught me how to ask myself really good questions.

This situation today is no exception. Based on the experience of how I responded after mum died, I've asked myself 'What are my beliefs now about death?'.

Given some emotional outbursts I had before, what kind of support might I need and what do I need to acknowledge? Where is my inner child and what might she need?

My love, life gives us difficult experiences. I just know you can navigate your way through this. Take time to tenderly ask yourself the questions you need. Everything will be ok.

DEVELOP AN ATTITUDE OF GRATITUDE

A friend announced that she was going to post daily on Facebook for a whole year. Her intention was to name what she was grateful for and she was inviting friends to join her.

To publicly post about my life? With honesty, no hiding, for 365 days? Urgh, I couldn't think of anything worse! Why would anyone want to read what I have to say? Isn't that just bragging? I wasn't sure I knew what gratitude really was. I worried I'd look stupid and of course, I'd have to show up for myself every day...I'd never manage that.

Yet for all my fear and freaking out, my heart told me to get out of my own way and get on with it. It was time to stop being a moaning Minnie and get some gratitude, from my heart. It was uncomfortable for the first three months, I worried all day about what to write. Was it superficial? Did I sound stupid? What should I post?

By March, I'd fully stepped out and was sharing the stuff my soul was made of. All my shadow side came out along with my gratitude for getting to know all the parts of me. I received beautiful emails from people, acknowledging my bravery for posting daily and how I reminded them to feel more gratitude. I was their daily reminder. Showing up daily had a positive impact on me and the wider community. It became infectious. Gratitude is a superpower, it can never be taken from you, it's yours alone and darn it feels good, so much better than complaining.

I invite you to gently place your hand on your heart, close your eyes and whisper the question: In this moment, what am I deeply grateful for? Gratitude is a feeling, invite emotion, love and appreciation into your whole being.

You are a beautiful soul, designed to feel the abundance around you, may gratitude in this moment bring you closer to your connection and your smile.

YOU ARE ENOUGH

I wasn't particularly gifted at school. I didn't have an attention span, I very rarely studied and my teachers never expected me to do well.

In junior school, our science teacher set a test on the topic of the planets. I poured my heart and soul into it! I loved this subject, it fascinated me. Fact and figures lodged with ease into my brain and with the help of our Encyclopaedia I learnt way more than my textbooks offered. On results day, the teacher walked down the classroom handing us our papers. She placed mine on my desk, I saw an A+, I was thrilled!

My teacher's comment was, "I don't know how you achieved this grade, somehow you cheated, I just don't know how". Instead of celebration, there was condemnation. This adult, my teacher, had a position of authority. Every day she had the choice of how to interact with the little people in her world. She could inspire or judge.

Today beautiful soul, forgive those who judged you poorly when you did your very best. Bring to mind some accomplishments that went unnoticed and celebrate them yourself. Acknowledge that you are enough, because you say so.

Hold depression with love

Today I'm grateful that I can talk about my experience of depression in public without shame. It was the loneliest and saddest time of my life. I masked it for years and never thought it would end. I couldn't imagine getting through it and I put a brave face on. Pretending was the most exhausting exercise I have ever participated in. I missed family weddings, get togethers, parties and simple cups of tea. I was unreliable and unable to speak up for myself. I hid away in embarrassment when what I deserved was love.

If you've opened this page, maybe you needed to hear this. I see you, I know your pain. As you sit here reading this, I am with you, I am gently whispering. My love, you are not alone. You are worthy. It's ok to relax your shoulders and breathe...give yourself permission to curl up under a blanket. You have everything within you to recover, take your gentle time.

What you need will be presented to you, so you can release the struggle. You are led and guided in every moment. Be willing to make friends with all parts of you, depression included. The precious child in you deserves your love and compassion, you deserve your love and compassion.

The Divine knows you are here and loves you. You are not alone.

It's your time to shine

By twelve years old, I was already a gifted athlete. I had the most incredible serve, that when executed with full technique and power, I'd score an Ace 90% of the time. My forehand was brutal and if I concentrated hard enough on form, so was my backhand. And...I could also play half-heartedly, so the ball would barely make it over the net.

One day, I'd made it to the final of my school tennis tournament. In front of the whole school, I flipped between powerful athlete and wet drip.

In my head, I was determined not to win, so...I pretended to do my best...while I threw the game. What a disservice to myself and my opponent. When she hit that final winning shot, my chest exploded with disappointment. I wanted to curl up and cry, I went home and did just that. Yet, I had invited that loss in and I never played tennis again.

This was a pattern but beloved, this pattern of not winning, not shining like a star, not stepping into our brilliance, it did not serve me, it does not serve you. You were a winner the moment you took your first breath of air. The Divine celebrated that day, knowing that a brilliant bright soul with so much potential had just stepped onto the planet.

You are enough. You are worthy. I invite you to work past your fear and step into your true self. It's your turn to shine as the universe intended.

PROCRASTINATION IS YOUR ENERGY COMING INTO ALIGNMENT

I can't tell you how many times I've told myself I'm a fabulous procrastinator, that I avoid making important decisions because I'm uncertain or weak. I was accused once of being 'flim-flam' by a colleague because I was unable to make, what I found, to be a really tough career decision and afterwards, they laughed at me.

It stems from my late Grandad. He used the words procrastination and prevarication daily. He usually directed them at himself but he said it about others too. I liked how the words rolled off my tongue, so I bought into the story that I too was a procrastinator and prevaricator. Those words haven't always been helpful though.

Consider this. The universe has to line up hundreds and millions of small details for our lives to manifest as we ask. Whilst we're in periods of indecision, the universe is creating magical alignment. The right people have to be in the same place as you, you have to hear a certain word or come across the right image, at the right time.

If, my love, it appears that you're struggling to make a decision, give yourself grace. Maybe the universe is still lining things up for you, maybe you're not ready to see the signs. It's ok to be in a period of deep consideration.

In times of uncertainty, I now say something different to myself. I say that my energy isn't aligned and that when it is, I will move forwards and it'll be obvious.

When your energy is aligned, you'll naturally take the action your soul desires. You will know what is right, when it is right.

"It's very important for the voices of women over fifty to be heard." says Gus. "To feel the strength and power in this age group, to change the cultural narrative of what it means to be a woman in midlife, is to set a new path for those women who follow".

Gus has found her clearest voice when dismantling the systems she doesn't want to be part of anymore.

Her voice as a mother, morphs as her children get older, she vocalises her desire for natural health and advocates for a reconnection to our intuition. Her latest role as post-menopausal woman, is where she feels she uses her strongest voice.

@gusgrima

GUS GRIMA

CONNECT TO THE CYCLES

I arrived in my forties not knowing that my body, my whole nature, was cyclic. Because of that, I worked against my body rather than with it. I overlaid the generic programme of how I was meant to operate in this world, rather than cultivating a sensitivity to myself and the way my body mirrored the natural world around me.

This especially showed up around menstruation, with ingrained messages like: keep going, hide it all costs, act like nothing's happening...basically 'don't listen to your body's needs'.

Ultimately, it made me both sick and unhappy and when I started to do the inner work of reconnecting to my stories, all the way back down the red thread to my first bleed, my mind was blown and everything shifted. The red thread is the story of your menstrual blood. Starting in puberty with your first bleed, ending at menopause with your last, it includes powerful, potent rites of passage, which most of us are completely unaware of. When not embraced, we can feel less and less empowered.

It's never too late to connect to your red thread journey, unpicking the stories, beliefs and thought patterns that were laid down when you got your first bleed about what it means to be a woman - you've carried those with you all your life!

Now I'm in that work, I see it's a pattern. Women arrive in their forties, disconnected from their bodies - way beyond how they look or nourish themselves - a fundamental separation from the wonder of their body's cyclic nature. We experience all four seasons in one month and across a lifetime, our energy changes in tune with the moon's twenty-eight-day cycle, even the twenty-four hour cycle is reflected in our life phases.

An invisible spiral of life that connects us so deeply, as women, to the natural world, we've come to live so separately from it, we've disconnected from the incredibleness of our bodies.

Cultivate a sensitivity to your body and the way it mirrors natures cycles. Start by paying attention to your menstrual cycle and how your body's needs change every day.

YOUR SENSE OF BELONGING STARTS WITHIN

For a large chunk of my life, I yearned for a sense of belonging, a place I felt at home. That feeling caused a lot of restlessness and dissatisfaction, I was always searching, seeking, I never felt settled, I didn't feel 'right'. I explored and tried many things, living in different places, making certain choices, not always logical but driven by a craving to find a more peaceful state.

Even when I lived with the love of a great man and the family we started, that feeling was there inside me. Wherever I was, I'd be thinking about where else I should or could live. I believed there was somewhere else I should be. Where I was, didn't feel like home.

In my forties, I made bold changes. I stopped using someone else's 'life user manual' and started using my own. As the years passed, I felt this sense of 'me'.

On reflection, I realised I was creating a sense of home and belonging within myself. I became the place I felt safe in, that I could return to, whatever was happening. I returned home to myself and with that, came peace.

You can scratch an itch by moving geographically - that can be a lot of fun - but if you're trying to fill an 'I don't feel at home' hole within you, you've got to cultivate a sense of belonging within your inner space, your heart. You have to get closer to and live, your true nature.

TIMING DOESN'T MATTER – IT'S THE JOURNEY

The funniest thing to me, is how much control I've tried to exert over my life. Ultimately, the big joke is that 'the timing of things will be what the timing of things will be!'. I don't feel we actually have much control over that at all. It's been one of the lessons to slap me around the face, over and over.

I've spent time hoping, wishing, striving and pushing to make things happen, then being disappointed or defeated when they didn't happen how I expected them to.

Now I try to sit back and watch my life like a movie. It's much more peaceful and relaxing than letting my mind get over-involved with all its plans and timelines! I've realised now that maybe some of those things I was trying to make happen weren't for me, maybe their timing wasn't right and I've noticed that in those times of pushing, I've lost out on moments of beauty that were right under my nose!

I was so whipped up into getting things fast, I missed the point. So...timing doesn't matter. What matters is the journey of life, the experiences of life and how we show up in each moment. It's the only moment that really exists and counts.

Have the courage to go slower. Take pauses in your day. Dance in the field of patience. It'll challenge you but it'll also bring you huge amounts of spaciousness and peace.

TRUST

There comes a point when you have to surrender to the unknown. I remember deciding to leave a big corporate job, making big, unsettling shifts in my business, taking my kids out of school to home educate them, initiating a home move out of the city and into the country.

Each time the decision to pivot came without having everything mapped out, without having any clear idea of the way through - simply starting with a knowing. Whilst we all crave security, safety and certainty, you can't be certain or sure about everything. You can't always get reassurance before you make a move. We never know if it'll turn out as we'd expected but we can trust.

Trust that uncertainty isn't necessarily a bad thing. Trust that when you walk with truth in your heart, anchored into an unexplainable knowing inside you, that becomes reassuring in and of itself. Trust also, that there are many potential unseen ways that something could turn out, not just the one you had in mind.

The mind has its plan, always...but life will unfold how it's going to, in weird and wondrous ways. You'll feel discomfort from time to time but learning to hold that discomfort and walk with trust in your heart anyway, is what makes you stronger.

When you lean into what's true for you and make moves from there, keeping an open heart and mind, you allow yourself to take the route that unfolds...with least resistance. Each route has its own twists and turns and you'll always, always learn something about yourself when you embrace each experience.

MASTER CONNECTING TO YOUR BODY AND YOUR INTUITION

The wisdom is within our bodies, not outside. Do you ever stop to tune into how your body is talking to you? Tension points, headaches, sore throats, tiredness...these used to be just a nuisance, I didn't see how I was a co-collaborator with my body, that we were meant to work together. Instead, I just pushed through.

My body speaks to me quietly too...the hunches, the knowings, the intuitive hits. Easier to miss if I'm wrapped up in 'but I said I'd do it!' mindset or too busy and overwhelmed with 'doing'.

My intuition speaks to me in the pauses, in the tiny moments of stillness I create within my family life. Quiet moments with myself early in the morning, tea or ceremonial cacao in hand. When I take deep breaths, walk in the woods or tune into the birdsong.

When I go slower and give my body what it needs, I climb down from my head and into my heart, I can hear the whisperings of guidance, little threads of gentle instructions: 'hold off doing that right now', 'what about this?', so subtle and easily missed.

The more I do this, the more I fall into a deeper and deeper trust of my body and intuition. Even when I'm navigating a challenging phase, everything feels calmer, simpler. A gentle hand of guidance on my back that I can soften into.

DON'T CARE WHAT OTHER PEOPLE THINK

"I don't care what other people think of me", was my first bold step in a new direction - on the path back to myself. At this point, I was in my mid-twenties and I'd lived with a deep-seated fear of what other people thought of me. I hid parts of myself, compromised myself and didn't express myself fully.

Fear of being judged, criticised or called out accompanied me from childhood into my young adult life. By my late twenties, I'd had my world shaken a little – the details aren't important – but by the time I was back on my feet, I decided to believe something else "I don't care what other people think of me".

I felt so much freedom as I integrated this into my life. I was choosing not to run my life by other people's (potential) opinions, judgements or expectations!

It was the first step back to my Self...and it led, over decades, to many more realisations about what beliefs, opinions and stories I held about me and the world around me, that simply weren't mine at all.

So, don't spend a lot of time worrying about what other people think of you. Follow your own compass.

FREEDOM STARTS WITH CLEARING THE CLUTTER

Freedom feels like a sense of spaciousness within me. And spaciousness comes from clearing the clutter from my inner space. Just like when a room or cupboard is cluttered, our inner space gets cluttered with 'musts', 'shoulds' and 'have to's'.

All the unconscious programming: what we think, our beliefs, expectations, the stories we tell ourselves – it takes up space. Examine some of that, are they your opinions or someone else's? If it doesn't resonate, chuck it out! Easy to say but it is possible to do.

Inner space also gets cluttered by over-attachment to our emotions and emotional reactions. I've spent days churning over something on a never-ending emotional rollercoaster, letting emotions run my day, make decisions for me, using my energy to suppress or deny them...wow...that cluttered up my inner space a lot!

So experience them and be present with your emotions but also take responsibility for them, rather than getting into blaming or shaming. Stop attaching too much drama to them. Let them pass through. It'll open up a sense of spaciousness within you, which for me, is directly linked to how much freedom I feel in my life.

WHEN YOUR BODY SAYS NO, ENOUGH IS ENOUGH

My body started talking to me through a set of health symptoms in my early forties. They bothered me enough to visit the doctors. It turns out those health symptoms were my body's way of saying 'Stop. This can't go on. You're changing and you cannot live disconnected from me anymore. There needs to be a change in pace around here. You need to stop doing things you don't like. Stop with the facade. Get real and honest about what isn't making you feel good. Pull your energy out of work and relationships that are exhausting you'.

I started listening instead of ignoring. I asked myself some difficult questions in the mirror and actually answered them with the truth!

I let the truth sink in. I reckoned with my life, where I was at and it was bloody uncomfortable! I wanted to look away, to stay numb. But I took a brave step and made the changes my body and soul were craving. I metaphorically took a match and started to burn down the things, patterns, stories and compromises that weren't serving me. I didn't know what I was doing! It was clunky AF. I didn't understand grace, I just took the first step - a massive one - stepping out of a well-paid career, to be at home with my babies. I knew it wasn't aligned anymore and that changing things was the start of the road back to myself.

When your body speaks to you, listen. Have the courage to make the changes it's asking of you.

The moment Martje read Lynette's
call for this book, her whole system
resounded with a decisive
'Yes, do this!'.

More women than she can
remember—strong, inspirational
figures—have spurred her to use
her voice and shaped her as she
grew older.

She nurtures the hope that every
woman who turns the pages of this
book will glimpse the wisdom of a
woman over fifty, absorb it into her
own life and find support,
encouragement and strength.

@martje.manthee

MARTJE MANTHEE

LEARN SOMETHING NEW EVERY DAY

When I got to school, I could already read. I'd taught myself and honestly, I really didn't understand why I needed to go. I quickly lost interest and motivation.

But when I'm really interested in something, it gives me the greatest pleasure to learn with dedication and ease. School really spoilt the joy to learn, it was many years before I rediscovered how fun it could be.

After nearly twenty years of working as an intensive care nurse, I came to a point where I thought there had to be more to life than just going to work every day. My job was very stressful and I lacked energy and enthusiasm. So, I started to look for something else and I found something that touched my heart immediately.

I always liked to take care of dying people and their relatives as a nurse and I found I could train as an End-of-Life Doula. I knew it would change my life.

There was no doubt or fear in learning something new and after a final exam following two years of study, I qualified. This was the beginning of several trainings which led me to being a hospice administrator. I never knew how much I loved learning new subjects, especially about personal development over the past few years.

I started a coaching qualification too and I'm grateful for this of the journey, it gives me so much joy to discover myself from a new perspective.

Learning is a gift! The older you get, the more important it will be to train your brain. Forget the old school days. Decide what you're interested in, there are loads of possibilities, do it your way.

FIND YOUR PURPOSE

To my mind, every human has a purpose in life, this is why we're here on this planet.

When I was young, socially, it was accepted that a woman's purpose was to have children and stay at home to take care of them. I never wanted children though, I'd ask myself again and again but there was this inner wisdom I felt that it wasn't my purpose.

So many times, I was asked about having children, especially by other women and my answer was often met with incomprehension! People just didn't understand. In my early thirties, I met my now ex-husband and the first thing he told me, was that he had five children. It didn't bother me at all, I always saw them as a part of him and they all still have a place in my heart. I called myself their 'bonus mum'.

Not being a biological mum, it took me a long time back then to find my own personal purpose. I found it though, I gave my wisdom, knowledge and empathy to people in need so willingly, I realised that this was my purpose...as a nurse, a hospice administrator and as a coach in the future.

Find your purpose, stay true to you, follow your heart and soul.

MENOPAUSE ISN'T AN ILLNESS

In my mid-forties, I was in a pretty bad state. I was sweating all night long, my sleep wasn't good and my mood scared me. I didn't recognise myself, I was angry, impatient, tired and exhausted.

'You're going through menopause. You can take hormones to feel better' my gynaecologist told me. I decided to try it with natural medicine and after a while, I felt better. Six years later though, on a long-awaited European trip, I developed severe muscle and joint pain...it took me a while to realise, these were menopause symptoms again! I felt so bad, that we halted our road trip and drove home.

I started my own research into hormones and realised that a healthy gut keeps hormones in balance and mine was not healthy! My preferred way of keeping my gut healthy now involves either four- or nine-day cleanses including Aloe Vera. This was a life changer; she is my daily medicine! I've fallen in love with this powerful plant.

Menopause is not an illness and we can nurture ourselves in this time of life. It's a stage every woman goes through, a new beginning actually, which we can invite in. When I realised I had menopause symptoms again, I was desperate and felt so alone, I had nobody I could talk to, I had to find my own way...you...my love, have this book!

I nurtured my body with healthy food and invited the menopause into my soul as a normal state, a stage of life I didn't want to fight against. From a spiritual perspective, it's been a new beginning, a chance to see myself from a new perspective.

It can be spiritual growth. Talk about your menopause to other women, you're not alone, we all grow together.

HOME IS SOMETHING YOU CARRY INSIDE

I've been looking for my roots all my life. I thought I'd find them in a specific place, a home town, somewhere that felt cozy and protected, where I would know everybody and the environment was familiar to me. But I didn't really have a home town. When people asked where I was from, I couldn't answer. We moved several times when I was a child, which always felt uncomfortable because I could never answer that question! I felt unrooted and lost sometimes.

As an adult, I moved many times too, I considered settling down in the Canary Islands or Australia. I still didn't know what I was looking for. I'd often ask myself questions like 'Where do I really come from?' and 'How does it feel?'.

Recently I found the answer. Home is inside me. I found a profound body-based form of Breathwork. It changed my life so much. When I heard about it, my whole system said 'Yes, I want to do this!'. I seemed to know it would heal my deepest wounds. And it did.

In one of those sessions, I found my inner home, there was no need for a special place in a geographical sense. You can be everywhere, if you feel at home in yourself. You are home. Always.

There are many ways to find your inner home. If you haven't found it yet, listen to your heart. I wasn't looking for a method or medicine, breathwork found me. If you listen carefully, you'll find what's right for you. Medicine is everywhere.

DISCOVER YOUR INNER CHILD

When I was a child, I sometimes wished I was a boy, not a girl. What I saw through the eyes of a child, was that boys are tough and nobody could hurt them, they didn't cry, they were strong. My father suffered from depression and being with him often felt heavy and sad, like a big heavy cloak laid upon the whole family. I thought I had to feel sad and depressed like him, I thought he expected that from me, I thought it was normal. But it didn't feel right.

I'd hear this inner voice whispering: 'If you were a boy, you'd be strong. You wouldn't be sad just because your father is, you'd be happy'. It was my little secret to protect me from the sadness around me. When I was on my own in my nursery, I imagined myself to be a boy and I felt lighter.

It took me many years to discover my femininity and vulnerability, I still had that little boy in me, who didn't want to be soft or vulnerable but when I understood why it was so difficult for me to open myself up, it felt like coming home. There are so many ways to discover and heal your inner child. See what feels right, it can absolutely change your life.

LET YOUR DREAMS BECOME REALITY

Two and a half years ago, while I was driving to work, I had a moment...I suddenly remembered I'd always wanted to buy a campervan and travel through Europe. At the time, my partner lived 100 km away, our dream was to live together but we hadn't worked out how. I had a vision...we could live together, quit our jobs, buy the van and cruise through Europe! "Why not do it?" I said to myself, my whole body said "YES!".

Fortunately, my partner said yes too and last year, our dream became a reality.   We started our journey in February. There have been several obstacles, a few fears to overcome and our road trip took a different turn than expected but it was completely worth it. Not for one single second have we ever regretted our decision. It's well and truly knocked off my bucket list!

Our time on earth is limited, so often we think we'll wait and do things when we're older but I've worked with the dying and the seriously ill for years, they taught me not to procrastinate - your dreams and wishes can come true.

So follow them! Let them come into reality and don't wait too long.

SELF-LOVE IS A MIRACLE

This is what most of us have discovered, when we've walked through life...that love from someone else, never replaces the love we need from ourselves.

When we fall in love, we get butterflies in our stomachs, everything is perfect! But love comes and goes...we break up with people, love hurts SO much, you might never want to fall in love again.

But humans strive for happiness and partnership. We need love to survive! I've fallen in love many times. I've been in three long term relationships and I was married for fifteen years. All those relationships I broke up, because I felt unhappy. But when I look back, I was unhappy with myself and I know I projected my own discontent onto my partners.

When I explored my own personality more deeply, I found out I didn't actually love myself! Honestly, loving myself with my whole heart has been a process and I'm still in it! On days when I feel unhappy and sad and getting mad at what my partner's doing wrong, I remember that I am loveable and I tell myself "I love you from the bottom of my heart". The feeling of love really is a miracle.

LISTEN TO AND TRUST YOUR INNER VOICE

For so long now, I've listened to my heart, I've found answers and wisdom there but I didn't always.

When I was younger, I'd look to others for my next right decision or choice. Other people always seemed more valuable than me. They always seemed to be so happy! I often wished I could be someone else, anyone other than me, I felt so empty and lonely, always fighting to be seen and to see who I really was.

When I put my hand on my heart, I remember all these instances. I remember how I'd look to others, sometimes in such pain and yet, I always had a feeling deep inside that I knew to be my own voice and I remember that resonating with my body and my heart.

I always knew that my inner voice had the answers really and when I listened, it gave me the trust that I was on the right path. And so today, I feel free, I can trust myself and my insecurities are gone. I stopped fighting against myself and accepted the woman who I am.

So, listen to and trust your inner voice. It will guide you like a compass through your life.

Tracey wants to remind every reader, "You are not on your own." Her enthusiasm towards the idea of writing her story here came from a desire to connect with other women, to share the trials and triumphs of her own journey.

She hopes to inspire others with her life experiences, to touch lives through her words, offering hope and perspective. This was her sacred intention in contributing to this shared reservoir of wisdom.

"I love being part of such collective wisdom which will help somebody at just the right time in their lives."

We think her words will make a significant difference to another woman's life journey.

@divineheartsholistichealth

TRACEY VAUGHAN

BEWARE OF GURU STATUS – TRUST YOURSELF

When I started my healing journey, I met the perfect teacher. She spoke to me in ways that touched my soul. She understood me. I was in awe of her and began nearly a decade of training with her.

The training resembled a kind of 'iron fist in a velvet glove' approach. I couldn't get enough of it though, I felt I was uncovering the real me. There was a small group of us who were all determined to work through our fears and unhealthy beliefs.

It was amazing. Until I reached a stage where I saw her for she really was. Human. We became equal. I no longer saw this enlightened guru in front of me. But a woman who had her own struggles. A woman who was trying to be the best possible version of herself. Boundaries were blurred, there were more demands rather than asks. I was finally understanding my authentic Self, so to then be asked to squeeze it into someone else's box was, of course, unacceptable.

I felt trapped. I couldn't speak about it to anyone in the group, in their eyes she was still on a pedestal. I had to leave. It was the hardest thing I've ever had to do but it strengthened my intuition and trust in myself. I found an inner voice and I'm not afraid to use it. I needed this experience. I'm blessed to have learned from it. I will always hold a space in my heart for my beautiful teacher but now I have my own tools.

Be wary of guru status. No-one is more superior or inferior than you. We may have our flaws but we also have our gems, we are human. Trust your intuition always.

LEARN BOUNDARIES AND ROUTINE

A typical Gemini, I love to flit from one idea and project to another. I've never been one for rules, spreadsheets or lists. I just go with the flow and see where it takes me.

Then along came Pippin.

I spent six months on the kitchen floor nurturing this beautiful little ball of fluff in the shape of a springer spaniel. After endless days of her tearing up the garden, ripping another pair of leggings and have me chase her around the house before bedtime, I thought 'what the fuck have I taken on!'.

My inner peace, house and wardrobe had been terrorised by her and I was at breaking point. I realised she was reflecting a lot of my own behaviours and that I had to develop some much-needed discipline. I needed structure. I needed boundaries. I needed a routine.

Now this may sound easy for some but these things were alien to me. I had to change and take responsibility for this little bundle of love, for the benefit of both of us. Everything I needed to get done was achieved between her needs. I became highly organised and focused on the day ahead, with a list of priorities.

This made life so much easier! I relax more knowing that walks, food, training and play all have their slots and I don't forget to schedule in some ME time. She's my greatest teacher. I've learned that you can still have fun whilst making lists!

IT'S NOT YOUR DRAMA, IT'S THEIRS

One of my biggest lightbulb moments was at the gym. Ironic really, because I dislike gyms but whilst marching on the treadmill, feeling irritation and frustration rise to the surface, it suddenly came to me…I felt like a parent to my parents!

I took a sharp intake of breath that almost choked me. I stopped the machine and just stood there, feeling a mixture of anger and relief. Then I burst into tears. I felt like the sounding board for them both, which left me emotionally drained.

Not only did I have my own feelings of confusion but I felt their frustration and disappointment with each other. I felt I'd turned into my parents' best friend, therapist and counsellor. But I didn't want that. I wanted to be their daughter. It was only when I really sat with my feelings that I discovered, they weren't mine. What I was carrying, was theirs.

I decided to give myself some space from them. I took myself out of the drama and let them battle it out on their own. I phoned them often but distanced myself until I understood that I didn't need to rescue either of them. They continued their drama, until they both went their separate ways.

Ever since that random thought in the gym. My parents and I have bonded in new way. We talk about our feelings, openly and honestly. We cry, laugh and have a new respect for each other. Even though that treadmill didn't get me anywhere physically, it certainly took me in a wonderful new direction.

IT'S OK TO BE SUPPORTED WHEN YOU NEED IT

I've always earned my own money. Ever since I was at school, my first Saturday job paid for a trip to the Caribbean with my aunt! I saved up and off we went. No debts to return home to and with my lily-white skin...no tan either!

From the age of seventeen, I was working and loving my independence. I didn't rely on anyone and financially was in a good place but at forty-six, I broke my ankle and had to stay off work. For the first time ever, I was in unknown territory both physically and financially.

I remember feeling so scared, because I had to do the one thing I had never done before: ask for help. It was awful. I saw it as a sign of weakness and it brought up a huge amount of defensive behaviour in me. My husband watched, wondering why it was so difficult for me to accept his generosity. I couldn't explain it but I sat with those feelings and breathed. I noticed where they were in my body. They were in my throat, chest and shoulders, I kept breathing and asked 'What message do you have for me?'. I recalled a memory, me as a child, comforting my mum.

And there it was. I wanted to protect others, I didn't want to add to their problems. I'd swallowed my own feelings rather than voice them in that moment and I'd learned to be self-sufficient! So, I whispered, 'It is safe for me to ask for help now?'. The answer was yes.

Being self-sufficient is important but so is asking for help when you really need it.

LOVE YOURSELF

Self-love is health love, it's time to put you first.
Self-love is wealth love, it quenches the abundance thirst.
Self-love means your love, that's given every day.
Don't wait for this love to come in any other way.

Self-love is not an external thing, that knocks upon your door.
Self-love is found deep within, the search is now no more.
It doesn't arrive for you to sign, like a parcel or a letter.
It's the little girl that resides in you, maybe you just haven't met her.

She's the one who may feel vulnerable, to be seen or even heard,
the one who responds to everything, even the unspoken word.
Self-love begins to awaken her; you birth her with your time.
Putting yourself before another, is neither selfish or a crime.

Self-love is the super power, that fuels your boundaries.
It gets easier to say no, than try and people please.
Check in with yourself love, tune into your heart so true,
now it's ready to be heard but it must first start with you.

So, invest in yourself love, it's the essence of your core,
by spending time on self-love, the universe gives you more.
You cannot fill the void love, unless it comes from you.
And any love that's left over, decide who to give it to.

NOTICE THE SIGNS YOU'RE BEING SENT

After thirty-one years in the airline industry, I finally hung up my wings. It felt right. I'd been talking about leaving and had been working as a complementary therapist alongside my flying. I was looking forward to doing the things I loved!

It was great! Not having a roster to live by, not getting up at three a.m, not commuting...bliss. I felt lost though. The pressure to 'earn' through my passion was weighing heavy and I was losing enthusiasm. I wasn't getting up until mid-morning, I was staying up late, watching utter crap on the tv and had the familiar feeling of depression setting in. I was spiralling. It took three signs for me to notice what I needed.

The first was a pigeon. It flew into the bedroom window with such a force, it died immediately, lying on the garden, it looked like a fallen angel. I cried. The second was a cat which ran past me with a bird in its mouth. I felt sad. The third was a bird drowning in a pond. I scooped him out, his little heart beating, he was trying to catch his breath. I cupped him to warm him up and sat there for forty minutes. He started to move, hopped onto the bench and into the bushes. I got home and bawled my eyes out.

I had made the connection. Birds. Wings. Flying. I needed to grieve. I needed to let go of this family I'd been a part of since I was seventeen. I had filed away intense sadness! I wept for six months, wrote about my feelings and let go, with love. Maybe you're being sent some signs you're yet to notice...

RECOGNISE YOUR MASK AND FIND OUT WHAT YOU REALLY NEED INSTEAD

I love all things funny. I grew up watching comedy duos and loved the slapstick. Humour ran in our family; we all had a PhD in sarcasm. This was how we displayed our love for each other: there were no hugs, no 'I love you', no encouragement, just sarcastic comments, piss-taking and put-downs.

And when we didn't get on, we'd have a 'dig'. A one liner. Delivered with such toxic fuel it was enough to go into space. This is how I learned to speak. So, I was stopped in my tracks one day when a lady I worked with tore a strip off me about my communication style. She did it graciously but I was stunned. I'd never had anyone question this before.

I reflected on it and felt terribly guilty. I apologised and we moved on but years later, I discovered my default archetype was the clown. I hated awkward silences and had to fill them with something, a joke, a noise, an impression. It was exhausting. I realised it was a mask I'd used to keep me safe, to show others that everything was ok and nothing bothered me. I learned to take that mask off. Every day, I'd look at myself in the mirror and genuinely say 'I love you' several times.

Just looking at myself was hard enough, I made a joke of the whole thing the first time I did it. I'd been using this mask in place of love. Pure love, from myself. Just looking in the mirror and seeing who that person was staring back was the biggest clue about how I showed up in the world.

The clown left the circus many years ago, which left me with some very big shoes to fill. And I did. With love, compassion, patience and grace for myself.

TRUST THE TIMING

Throughout my life I never had the desire to have children. Some people found it so odd that I didn't have this maternal instinct, they proceeded to remind me of the time left on my biological clock.

It was interesting watching people's reactions to my decision, which usually caused them to go off on a tangent! I've always been open and honest about it and never understood what all the fuss was about.

I had never met anyone I wanted to settle down with enough to even have such a conversation about having kids but at forty-one, when I was in a good place, mentally, emotionally and spiritually, I made the decision to spend my life with someone. He swept me off my feet, he was nine years younger than me, with an eight-year-old son.

That wasn't part of my plan and actually I couldn't bear the idea of being a stepmother, even the word filled me with dread but I wasn't going to give up on a wonderful relationship just to avoid stepping up. Hell no.

I believe this was all part of the divine plan for my growth and maybe the reason I'd never had children before, because I was going to be blessed with one later in life, when I had the wisdom and love to offer. The timing was perfect.

The universe knows exactly what we need and when to deliver it. Some things we wish for may not arrive in the way we expected but we must still see it as a gift.

Accept that you are open and ready to receive.

You are open
and ready to receive

The warrior woman in Elaine has led her to speak for the underdog many times in her life. From the playground, to her career in the television industry and on stage, she's put herself in the firing line and spoken out against the web of control and manipulation coming from those 'in power'.

"I'm happy to put controversial ideas out on paper" she says, "as a freelance journalist, I fear that free speech is being slowly eradicated from our world. Ultimately to bring change, one must keep an open mind and not to judge too quickly."

We hope that Elaine's conviction for free speech will inspire you to use your words to stand up for what you believe in.

@hillisticyoga

ELAINE HILL

TRUST THAT YOU ARE CONNECTED AND SUPPORTED

I believe that everything and everyone is connected. The birds, the seas, the man across the street - all like drops of water in this vast ocean of the Divine. I see us all as extensions of ourselves, fractals of the Divine; trying to keep our heads above water to varying degrees of success. I feel my life experiences are expressions of the Divine passing through me as I journey back to Source. A contract of lessons and liberations for the soul growth I agreed to embody in this earthly realm. Remembering this, tames the blame game in me and allows forgiveness to flow a little easier.

It's taken a long time and much spiritual seeking to deeply feel this truth in my waters. Like a slow osmosis, this 'seeping in' of knowledge that every person or obstacle on my journey has been my teacher or a reflection of what I've projected, has helped me set the right course of action. I truly believe that what I put out comes back through this sea of connected energy, together with initiations to master.

Bathing in the knowing that I am a small yet integral part of this grand design, is both awe inspiring and humbling. Trusting that my soul is supported, learning, loving and experiencing this ocean of connected energy, helps to remove fear and anchors me.

So trust...trust that you are connected and fully supported.

SLOW DOWN, ENJOY LIFE MORE

Looking back on my early life, I rushed my way through much of it on a mission to prove myself. I smashed goals at breakneck speed as though time was running out.

My ego was looking to leave a legacy. Catalysts such as the bully teacher who marked my card with 'could do better' and the feminist zeitgeist proving that women could break that glass ceiling, fuelled my need to achieve.

Like the proverbial bull in the china shop, allowing my masculine side to dominate, I had simply missed the point, looking in all the wrong places for approval and my reason to be. The birth of my children was the revelation. They taught me to relax and view life with the wonder it deserves. They reminded me of the virtue of patience and the need to nurture my own inner child.

I could slow down and appreciate every now moment, delighting in their achievements with praise, rather than chalking them up like a badge of honour to myself. I do not seek approval anymore - I realised that's a programme not of my making.

Taking my time, embracing my softer feminine side has been the best decision. There's a lot to be said for the continental habit of sitting in a cafe and watching the world go by. Life isn't about the end goal but enjoying the journey along the way at a much more enjoyable pace.

RECOGNISE THE MATERIAL STUFF FOR WHAT IT REALLY IS

I've always wanted to NOT want what I really don't need. It's nice to have lovely things but I've felt at times the more I had, the more I wanted. Desire seems to be a black hole, there's always more to want.

It's an illusion though, cast by the powers that be who own and control everything money orientated. Their media and marketing, from inception, have played a blinder; keeping our focus on the material (external) rather than the spiritual (internal).

I feel they've preyed on our individuality and creativity, bringing unhealthy competition and division, topped with a spiral of debt. They've programmed our lifestyles and even put a value on what jobs deem us worthy.

As a freelancer most of my working career, I always had to be careful with money. I could want but not have most of the time. Now as I see through the illusionary spell, I pause and breathe when that devil of desire arrives at my door and decide from my heart, not my head, whether that latest bauble's shine is really worth its weight in gold.

HEAL WITH MOTHER OCEAN

I love my relationship with Mother Ocean. I can't believe I was brought up by the sea and was hardly ever in it. As a girl, I loved mermaids and seashells and books about the ocean, I swam all the time in the local swimming pool. Had I lived somewhere warm, I'm sure I'd have lapped up daily dips like warm soothing showers.

After twelve years of living in London, my love of the seaside lured me back home to the east coast of Scotland. One hot, sunny day, my kids and I went to the beach and they dared me in for a swim.

My inner child actually jumped at the challenge and I haven't looked back since! I love the feel of that cold water as it glides over my skin, it's a shock to be sure but the power of the waves and the swell of the current thrills as much as it chills.

It's an intoxicating addiction that leaves a warm, fuzzy feeling. Wild swimming brings out the wild woman in me, either that or I'm just a crazy old lady, I really don't know but I'm so glad I gave it a go! It makes me feel 'on it' for hours afterwards. It's known to be good for mental health and raging menopausal hormones - it certainly sorts the hot flushes out. It grounds me in the same way that standing barefoot on the grass in the sun does. Instant healing given freely from Mother Ocean herself. What joy!

TURN A MOTHER'S GUILT INTO GRATITUDE AND ONE-ON-ONE TIME

It was an arrow to the heart and the tears came. A perfectly normal day, I'd just dropped the kids at school and was clearing the breakfast dishes when Abba's 'Slipping Through My Fingers' came on the radio. My mother used to play it on her record player while doing the housework. Nostalgic feelings of that precious time with my mother, mingled with guilt as the 'sand in my hour glass' was sifting fast with my own children.

Precious time slipping away as I busied myself with so many other things. I've often felt a gut punch from a mother's guilt. My love for my kids is profound, it defies measure, save the cruel restraint of the time we can tuck them under our wings. But guilt is such a low vibrational emotion which deserves no place in a loving mother's heart.

The tears dried though when the guilt transformed into gratitude. I was blessed, raising three beautiful, funny, independent beings who cared about the world. As my mother raised me, so I was raising my own.

When feelings of guilt niggle in, I carve time with my kids one-on-one. Undivided attention before bed to listen about their day or take them for a walk. A chat goes a long way. I tell them often how much I love and am proud of them. It's the little things that make the most difference, help them feel valued and are easier to slot into a hectic life.

When my children do leave my every day presence to forge their own path, I hope they'll deeply feel their mother's blessings and delight for a job well done, as I do for my own.

LOOK INSIDE YOURSELF FOR THE ANSWERS

Digital fatigue is most definitely a thing, people cling to their smart phones like a life raft in a sea of information overload and that often brings anxiety.

It's knowledge exhaustion and it comes in other guises too. I've hoarded mountains of books in my life, I used to have at least ten books on the go, such was my voracious search for the meaning of life or worse...how to become the best version of me and all that rubbish!

I was a self-help book junkie in my twenties and thirties. As I matured, my book addiction moved to those on raising babies which created nothing but angst and guilt together with a huge dollop of OCD! I sterilised everything within an inch of its life but thankfully, by child number three, I was over that, along with all the books!

In my forties, I read about ancient truths, the knowledge and the wisdom of indigenous people. Simple and frankly common-sense advice, I discovered that living life 'well' isn't rocket science, I was doing it already, the answers were within myself and my intuition. Simplifying life and watching the world go by, it turns out, was the key to my happiness!

So now in my fifties, I've stopped looking outside for the answers, instead I look to the wisdom within. I've found a space in my heart where I visualise my connection to my God/Self and I ask my questions there, trusting what comes.

I still keep the books on my bookshelf...I may not have got 'here' had I not gone 'there'! But for those still in the sea of self-help books or clinging to their smart phone life raft looking for guidance, remember life is about living right 'now' without fear.

Enjoy all that floats by in full technicolour and take ownership when required. You know the answers are within you already, so use your wings and soar.

THIS IS YOUR CALL TO THE WILD!

The clarion call, the sound of the unsung hero, a call to the wild and a whisper back to the Mother, the Divine Feminine may have been long shrouded in mystery but she is not lost. The strength of her whisper carried to women everywhere, a message that rings true to the hearts of all who hold her dear. I want to say to all the women who read these words 'rise and be heard'.

Your song is strong and worthy. Never forget the beauty of the maiden within, the love of the mother you are to all around you and the wisdom of the crone you will be or have become.

A message from one woman to another...

Show up every day, with your head held high.

Face the trials of life, if they arise.

I salute you!

You are outstanding!

Bring out your joie de vivre
and make your raison d'être a promise to never hide your light under a bushel for anyone!

I've learned that the only way to live authentically, is to honour the good bits and the not-so-good bits of myself with acceptance. If we are so 'fearfully and wonderfully made', then are we not perfect just as we are? Sing your song loud and proud darling, shine like that beacon of light beckoning all those weary women home, until we are a choir of heavenly angels arising in balance once more.

This is your call to the wild!

STAND IN YOUR POWER

In my early twenties, I travelled the world with my job as a television presenter for a holiday show. In awe of all the attractions and people I met, it was such an enlightening experience. When visiting Asia one time, we arrived with all our film equipment and the relevant documentation but getting through customs was problematic. Some negotiation was required and I was deemed the best person for the job! The officials were harsh, armed with guns and to say I was a bit scared, was an understatement.

The warrior woman in me was activated on full though and eventually we passed through. Days later, while we were filming, I sat outside a beautiful temple learning my script when I was tentatively approached by some small children, it took them a while but eventually they touched my arm and squealed in delight.

I was perplexed but laughed with them. I'm not sure if they thought I was real or not. I was blonde, dressed in white - did I seem to them like a ghost? Then their mothers approached me, pointing at their lips and mine. I understood immediately and I reached inside my bag, gifting them the lipstick I was wearing!

They were so grateful, I was so humbled, tears flowed. For so long, women have soldiered on through thick and thin, giving to all (except themselves), yet the call of the feminine and her beauty is strong.

If that shade of colour on their lips made them feel defiantly beautiful, I felt so honoured to have played a small part in that. It's a scene I have never forgotten. And so, I say to women the world over, standing in your power takes many forms whether it's using your wit or your war paint, don't forget to bring that beauty within out!

Support your sisters, for together we rise and become some force indeed.

A mother to three treasures, two
boys and one girl, Andrea is inspiring
them every day to speak their truth
by speaking her own. She says it's
"an inner truth" that
she is guided to share.

An artist now, she is leaving an
indelible mark on those who meet
her through her creativity, her
dedication to love and her appetite
for living life on her terms.

Andrea had never written before this
book but it resonated with her so
deeply, she knew she had to take
part. Allow her powerful words and
energy to sink into your being and
find your own courage to thrive.

@andreaolafs_andartica

ANDREA FÁFNIS ÓLAFS

CONFIDENCE IS KEY

To me, it has been a pleasant realisation to discover that life got better and better as I grew older and bolder. When I was younger, I assumed that life would be a declining experience. But on the contrary and to my surprise, it got better!

The thing about reaching my age, is the privilege of having enough experience and wisdom to see that each decade has new learnings. The more confidence I've had to challenge myself and take on new experiences with open arms, the more confidence I've gained.

Believe me, I've pushed myself many times out of the comfort zone, travelled without a plan, moved abroad a few times and had children. I've been a manager, a leader of a big organisation, speaking publicly and in the media, I even ran for both the presidency and parliament in my country! It's also been important to me to remember, that after each episode of a downturn, there's been another upturn that has brought great appreciation and gratitude.

We are creatures of habit but most of us also need variety and new challenges every now and then. That's how we grow and learn and most of us like to grow and learn. If you know yourself to be an explorer, be confident enough to travel the world! Live in different places, get to know different cultures.

Remember you're not a tree, you are not stuck, you can move. Don't plan ahead too much, don't be too rigid - let your path reveal itself by being open to new places, changes of course and different options. The key attitude for making these kinds of things happen is confidence - JUST DO IT!

'TO BE OR NOT TO BE', MAKE A PACT WITH SOURCE

Most people have to ask themselves, at one point or another, the question; 'to be or not to be'. It can relate to a situation in life, a relationship, a job etc or it can relate to life itself.

Life, at times, can become overwhelming, empty and painful to the point that some feel as though leaving it is their only answer.

If you ever find yourself in this vibration or situation, I would invite you to allow this page to light a little spark within you, a little spark of curiosity. Because curiosity, I believe, is a true life spark and it can be enough to bring hope to the Soul. I encourage you to make a pact of some sort with Source, to ask for guidance and direction, to listen attentively to the world around you, to all the little cues that may come to you. Follow them, trust that it's your guidance from Source.

They might come to you as just little things that give you little insights - or they might come as huge revelations. Perhaps an elder will ask you when you last sang and danced, maybe someone will speak about true love, maybe you'll come across knowledge of how someone else felt the same as you and what the cause was. Maybe someone will share their healing method and it'll ignite curiosity in you, to follow that path too.

I myself had been suffering from unexplained ill health from long-term and repeated exposure to toxic mould. I got seriously ill, I hadn't realised how dangerous it could be. I asked Source for guidance and I received and accepted the guidance for many different healing methods, alternative healing and even a shamanic healing journey which has all helped tremendously.

Make a pact with Source, that you'll attempt to write a new chapter for your life and then start walking. Start walking and the path will appear.

TRY NOT TO JUDGE

Oh my god, even just thinking about writing this is bringing tears to my eyes. But I know I must. As a result of my own experiences, I feel a responsibility to protect how people who take their own lives, are thought of. Please be careful with your words. Do not judge. Remember, you are not in their shoes and you didn't know how they felt. No-one knows their desperation or their abyss.

Their decision will not have been an easy one. Their conclusion, that death would ease their pain, will have been hard beyond measure. So many seem to feel like suicide is selfish but I believe it's a lack of self-love. You see, being lost for a long while and maybe repeatedly during a lifetime, in some kind of depressed state, whether it's a state of loss or grief, a state of pain inside the heart and soul, a state of no purpose or a state of nothingness, simply takes its toll. And often, it's so hard to detect.

People become very adept at smiling, being loving and friendly, even when they don't feel a connection or love inside of themselves. People about to commit suicide go out, they travel, socialise and work. Their emptiness is hidden and becomes bigger and if you've never felt a sense of any of that, please don't pretend you understand, it's ok to admit that you don't, just don't judge. Let's remember them with love and compassion.

ASK FOR PERMISSION

In my younger years, I was always very blunt. I've been very honest if someone asked me about something, I never lied to them, I told them what I considered to be true. And I've always been an empath, eager to help people if I can. As I grew older, I became more cautious. The years taught me that people didn't always want my advice or opinion on what they were going through, sometimes, they just wanted me to listen while they spoke. They were simply trying to formulate how they felt or maybe to understand their own feelings by speaking out loud.

Whether I advised them or not, people trusted me with their deepest secrets, sometimes very heavy stuff. So, I decided to start asking for their permission to share what was coming to me as I listened to them. I started to ask if they'd be ready to listen, even if it might be difficult to hear.

By asking for and gaining their permission, I felt I was able to alleviate the pain from their harsh reaction as I spoke a difficult truth or asked them to consider a different perspective. Today, I even go as far as to ask people if they really want my advice, knowing that I might have a different option. I ask them to contemplate whether they really want to change anything or if they'd rather keep the status quo.

Either way, I've found asking permission before giving any advice opens up the other person and softens how it's received. So, since you're reading this, I ask your permission to let my words enter your mind and allow them to resonate with you for contemplation.

THE G-SPOT

I actually never thought I'd be sharing anything as private as this but it came as a flash into my headspace when I was prompted and I decided to go with the flow. I'm one of those women who didn't fully discover that tiny little pleasure spot (that gives and gives and gives!) until after I'd gone through a long period of shamanic healing, followed by meeting new love at the age of forty-seven.

You see, it wasn't big but finding it was! I think it's the same for many women, I wasn't able to open this part of myself up fully until I was with a partner I trusted, not only with my body but with my soul, heart and whole being. When I felt secure enough to be myself and felt totally adored and loved, I found it. I've heard women who say they still believe it's just a myth that it isn't really there...but it is and with the right touch, we can feel its incredible power.

Explore this area, inside your body, yourself and with your trusted partner. You might not necessarily feel it through intercourse but the right finger touch will find it. I can't tell you exactly how, that's for you to find and explore but take time to learn about this important little spot and open yourself up to its unending pleasures!

HIGHER LOVE

My separation was a devastating time. I felt very guilty for breaking up the family and for a while, I felt like my life was over. I still remember something one of my divorced friends said, "There is life after divorce," he said, "it will get better. You just have to get through this part, the grief and the sorrow".

Now, I want to make sure that by sharing this, I'm not advocating for or recommending divorce. On the contrary, I always encourage people to work on their differences if possible. But sometimes it simply doesn't work.

During the time of my separation, I was hanging on to a very thin thread of hope and actually, when I was by myself, I really didn't feel any hope at all. I felt like life was over. I didn't want to go through the roller coaster of a love relationship again and there really wasn't much that gave me joy or hope, except my children.

One day, I decided to pray through the song 'Higher love' by Whitney Houston which strongly resonated with me. Each time I sang that song in my car, turned up very loud, I was speaking out to Source. I was clearly stating that I didn't want to be here for the same kind of love again, that I wanted a higher love, that I would open up my heart only if I could get to the 'next level'.

A few weeks later, I met someone SO unlike my ex...the complete opposite and right from the start it felt 'next level'. We are both loving so much stronger and deeper than before, surrendering fully. Yes indeed, there is life after divorce and in my case it's filled with joy and love and a much more fulfilling relationship.

Love is there for you, ask the universe for it...sing it...pray for it...speak it out loud! The universe always hears. Listen to the answer.

WHERE IS YOUR JOY?

I truly believe that adulthood makes some of us forget or lose our joy, our inner knowing of what we really love so much, that we can lose ourselves in for hours on end.

I did. I was so distanced from my inner child, I'd forgotten the things that brought me joy. During one very dim place in my life, I asked Source to show me or guide me towards, feeling just a little bit of joy.

I was so low I could hardly feel any joy at all. I believe it was the Goddess of Art who came to me in a dream and said to me in a motherly way that I would find my joy if I simply played with colour. She didn't tell me to paint outright, I think she probably knew I'd have just dismissed that with an 'I can't paint' statement.

A couple of years passed before I finally got it! Prompted by a new love in my life, flying high on love, I started painting. And when I did, I remembered that dream!

Such tremendous joy flowed through me, constant happiness...allowing me to be in a pure flow of creativity and just paint.   Now I paint almost every day and I exhibit my work.

When people around me are a little bit down, I ask them to close their eyes and go back to childhood and find what it was they enjoyed the most. It's still there – it just needs to be brought out fully and embraced.

If you experience this loss of joy for long periods in your life, maybe it can help you too to ask Source for insights, to guide you towards the joy of your soul. Answers can come to you in many different ways, through dreams, intuition, direct prompting from other people. Remember to listen.

HOLD YOUR BABIES CLOSE

I never knew how much I would regret 'training' my babies not to cry or need me during the night. I was thirty back then and advised to see a 'sleep specialist' for children, so my little baby boy wouldn't need to cling to me during the night. I followed her advice. My son did finally learn to sleep on his own but it took a long time to 'train' him and it felt painful for both of us

A decade later came son number two, I decided I'd start early with him and around his sixth month I attempted sleep 'training'. He cried so deeply. He looked at me with sad and broken eyes almost as if asking, 'Why are you doing this to me?'.

When I looked long enough and deep enough into his eyes, I knew. My motherly intuition told me it was all wrong and that it was simply much safer and better for my child to be held in my arms, to lay his ear and head on my chest and be in my warm cuddle.

Connecting to your children is so vital for their health and growth, there's usually a good reason for their crying...something is bothering them. Maybe they have tummy ache, maybe you're eating something that's upsetting them through your breastmilk, maybe environmental mold toxins or maybe they simply need touch, body warmth.

They need us. They need to be with us. A long time ago I read that research showed young children start producing high levels of the stress hormone cortisol when they're away from their parents for more than six hours at a time.

They don't necessarily show any sign of stress immediately but the body is giving them the stress signal. Hold them close my love – for you and for them.

"I feel that women's voices are more valuable than ever, if we are to leave our daughters a legacy"
says Alexandra.

Her mother was the inspiration for her in finding her voice and now, she is that for her children. As her daughter's biggest advocate, she speaks out for the right to inclusion and support for children with special needs.

Her wish is for her chapter to reassure women that they are not alone, to reach out to their sisters in the wider world and to create ripples of support everywhere.

@maya_holistic_therapies

ALEXANDRA FRASER DURAN

YOU ARE ABSOLUTELY UNIQUE

I was born in a place where education was very important. An average student, I struggled with school really, I don't have any good memories from those times. Everyone in the family looked and seemed so much smarter than me but I did have a great imagination and I liked to play. I loved music, dance and theatre and I had a great memory.

I often memorised long poems and used to recite them, I wanted to become an actress and in spite of my shyness, I did things I never thought I'd do. I went to castings and put myself out there.

I was interviewed to celebrate my twenty-second birthday on TV in Barcelona...in Catalan. It was incredible, I was asked to recite a poem, I talked about my country of origin, my linguistic abilities and adapting to a new country. I danced too.

That moment for me was the start of believing in myself. For a good month or so afterwards, people who had watched the program congratulated me and were inspired by my words. I always stood against injustices, I realised that I'd had an opportunity to create change by simply being me and speaking my own truth. I realised my path was not in academia but in doing the things I loved most... dancing, writing poems in Spanish, learning languages, travelling and following my own intuition my own unique path. In that moment everything changed.

You are absolutely unique, try to stop comparing yourself to others.

SAYING GOODBYE TO YOUR LOVED ONES, HONOURING DEATH

Growing up in a family where reincarnation, past lives, tarot, astrology and psychic surgery were everyday discussion, I created my own way of being, feeling and believing in the afterlife. I became acquainted with words such as spirit, mediums, healing and death.

My grandfather died when I was six years old and I knew he'd gone home. He was no longer with us and while some people were very sad, I knew he was fine. Then I lost my Grandmother, she was so close to me and came to visit me before she passed. We were living very far apart but I knew she was passing through, I said thank you for everything and in a second, she was gone.

By the time it was my mum's turn, at the young age of sixty-nine, I'd experienced great loss and I knew this one was going to be a particularly hard one. She was everything to me. We spent days talking about how she would come back and visit me as a butterfly and how she'd always look after us. She chose when to go and how. She became aware of her mum near her, coming close to pick her up. She smiled, shed a tear and she was gone.

I thanked mum for the open conversations about death and dying. Knowing it, helped me understand this process. We all held space for her in a beautiful circle of light. Death is part of being human. We're here, on this earth, just passing through and in a split second everything can change. When we open a door to these discussions it can ease the pain. Death is simply a new rebirth back home where we reunite again with our loved ones.

Be open to conversations so that when the time comes, you're able to honour death as another rite of passage in life.

THE UNEXPECTED IS A GIFT

The news of a little girl made us really happy. And then the unexpected happened. We were told she had Down Syndrome. My husband withdrew and distanced himself for a little while. I understood. We all need different ways to process the unexpected. Mixed emotions rushed through me, I became a fierce tigress, I wanted to protect her at all costs. I wanted her to feel loved and accepted no matter what.

The unexpected can break our hearts for a time. But, with time, it can also break us open to new possibilities, possibilities greater than ourselves.

By the time we had our daughter, we realised that her quirks, her traits, were not mistakes after all. She was uniquely created and uniquely loved by Source and by us, in fact, by all who knew her name.

We thought our lives were ending when we got this news. Instead, we got a new beginning. The gift of her presence, her innocence, her joy and her uniqueness has opened our hearts to depths we'd have never seen or felt otherwise.

If the unexpected has landed at your door, close your eyes, take a deep breath and ask your heart to guide you and give you the tools to navigate the 'new' from a higher purpose. You can always respond from a place of love rather than fear.

IT'S OK NOT TO BE OK

I lost both my prematurely born daughter and my mum in a short space of time. And in that process, I lost myself too. Grief is such a powerful emotion; it comes to your door without permission. It felt like being swallowed by a gigantic wave...drowning.

I continued to move through life despite the pain, others needed me to love them and I did. But one day a friend asked me how I was. There was a pause and my eyes started watering, she then said, "It's ok not to be ok you know!". In that moment I cried and cried and cried.

My own tears eventually lifted me through to the surface to a lighter path, where I was able to breathe and appreciate the warmth sun on my skin. I'd been shattered and I was now seeing parts of me coming back to my body slowly.

I realised I'd been holding so much tension and I wasn't allowing the pain to rise and be seen and be heard. My friend gave me permission with her words to release all of that.

I held myself with tenderness and compassion as I weathered the storm. My tears and my rage were welcomed, along with the joy and the laughter. In that moment, I understood the message, 'it's ok not to be ok' and with that, everything started to shift.

TRUST YOUR INTUITION

I knew I'd been cheated on but my brain kept saying, 'He would never do that!'. My gut and inner knowing knew I needed to exit this relationship but I was hanging onto something I thought mattered.

I ignored the red flags, the signs and the feelings. I chose not to see them. Six months later, a friend visited me at work. We exchanged looks and, in an instant, I knew the truth. He was the husband of the woman my partner had been seeing. I saw the pain in his eyes. We both cried, it was time to leave him. I said no more.

That was the last time I tolerated such things. From that moment on, I trusted my intuition one hundred per cent! From feeling like the victim of betrayal, I became my own hero.

Don't dismiss the signs.

THE PAIN YOU'RE CARRYING MIGHT NOT BE YOURS

I was born with my umbilical cord around my neck, I was blue when I entered this world and as a child, I seemed to know that. I remember behaving as though I had nothing to say.

It felt like my voice wasn't important and I spent my teenage years, right up till my twenties, pleasing others, never speaking up for myself.

I wanted to feel seen and heard, in fact, I moved away from home at a very young age in order to find my own voice. I'd been aware of some repetitive patterns in my relationships and I'd felt a huge sadness at not being seen or understood.

At some point, I realised, a lot of the pain I was carrying wasn't mine to carry. I had a light bulb moment when I turned twenty-seven. I suddenly saw and felt the heaviness I'd been carrying and realised it wasn't mine but memories of loss and pain from my mother's side.

In that moment I started to shed layers and layers of conditioning and sadness. As I began to walk my own path, I began to find my own voice, my own unique tune, unshackling myself from my mother's wounds, healing the ancestral path.

Now, when I tune in to myself, when I feel heavy or sad, I ask, 'Is this mine or someone else's?'. And in that moment I trust.

DON'T LISTEN TO ANYONE ELSE, FOLLOW YOUR INSPIRATION

There have been many times in my life when people have said 'Don't do it!'. When I dreamed of living in Paris and learning French, people thought I was crazy and I went anyway, without knowing any French at all.I went for a job as a bartender there when they'd already fired the last girl because she hadn't spoken French. But there I was, a Colombian girl with a smattering of English and absolutely no French and still I landed the job! They gave me three months to learn the language and fast forward a year, I was in the middle of beautiful Paris, in charge of the whole place!

Don't listen to anyone else, follow your own inspiration, say YES to things that inspire you and bring you joy. Don't ever let anyone make you feel you can't!

FIND CONNECTION FROM A NOMADIC LIFE

I come from a family of Nomads. I was born in Colombia, we moved a lot but a massive move came when I was thirteen years old...to Spain. A new continent!

The same language but with different ways of saying and doing things, I had to learn Catalan to enter their school system and that was so very different. Despite that, I made new friends and adapted relatively easily. By twenty, I'd been to seventeen schools!

It was at twenty-five, I moved to France and by the time I was thirty, I spoke five languages. These massive life changes taught me to learn quickly...about different cultures and their languages, to become chameleon-like! I learned to adapt to new environments, to blend and to add my own personality into the mix and while it wasn't always easy, I realised that no matter where you come from, everyone wants to be loved and accepted within a community.

We all want to connect with other people in ways that touch our hearts, we're here to support and help each other in the best possible ways. No matter where you are, your tribe will find you!

A daughter and a sister, Marjolein
has used her voice clearly and with
authority in her career.

She wanted to write a book and let
her request be heard by the
Universe. Not long after, she saw
Lynette's call-out and she knew this
was her chance to put pen to paper.

She hopes her reader will know that
life has more in store for them than
sadness and struggle but that
sometimes that's a necessary part of
finding and enjoying the deepest and
most satisfying of
rewards in life.

"Never give up hope!" she says.

@leintje_2410

MARJOLEIN RUITER

KEEP YOUR HUMOUR, IT REALLY SAVES THE DAY

As a child I laughed a lot, especially during my stay at Curacao from the age of three until nine. Life was heaven for me in the Caribbean, always sunny and warm, a free life, going to the beach often.

When I was nine, we moved back to the Netherlands and from there, life became more serious. I was intimidated by the Netherlands: so many people and so loud! Life was faster and my 'problems' began.

I was bullied, I had all sorts of health issues: allergies, bowel disease and breast cancer. I had so many deep conversations with my mother during that period. Sometimes we'd fight, even over the phone, it showed how hard it was for me as a young woman but for my mum, all those worries! Even when we fought though, we'd use humour; we'd never hang up the phone without a laugh, for us it was a way to connect, to make things a little less heavy than they probably were. It kept us going.

I always try to keep it lighter with humour, it's like the sun comes out for a bit. In dark days, it's sometimes hard to find the humour. But if you really try, you can always find something to laugh about, it helps!

YOU'RE GOOD ENOUGH AS YOU ARE

Growing up and almost ready to go to primary school, my dad let me believe that every child should have lost at least one milk tooth before starting school. He was a really sweet man, it was a joke but all summer, I did my utmost to lose my first tooth. Unfortunately I failed.

I interpreted this as not being good enough for school. I felt like I let my parents down, I felt really powerless and for a very long time, I believed I wasn't good enough. As a teenager, the girls told me I wasn't good enough, I was too fat apparently, I wasn't funny, I wasn't a good friend...my first boyfriend even broke up with me because 'I wasn't good enough!' and he broke my heart!

It's only been so recently that I've realised, through working with a Wellness Coach, that everyone is good enough, even with their flaws.

My love, look yourself in the mirror and tell yourself 'I am good enough!' Let that become your normal. Keep reminding yourself: you are good enough, you are good enough, you are good enough as you are.

BE TRUE TO YOURSELF

During my childhood, people often told me that what I thought or said was 'only in my head'. They meant that no-one else thought what I said was true or held any value, that it was just true in my head. Due to this, I doubted myself for most of my life. It had a big influence on what I said, what I wanted and what I thought.

A couple of years ago, I spent a lot on time of my own and for the first time, I experienced peace and quiet. My world stood still. At first, it felt very confronting and scary but later, I discovered I liked the quietness and the peace, there was room for my own thoughts and opinions: what was important to me. I realised I hadn't been true to myself for my whole life!

I also realised it was time to start. I started by reading a lot about the human mind and spirituality. I listened to loads of podcasts and with every book and every podcast, I realised I was growing, finding out what I loved, what my thoughts on subjects really were – without the confusion of someone else's opinion or being told that they were only true in my head!

And now at fifty years old, I can honestly say, I am finally true to myself and it feels so good. I will now always stay focussed, so as not to drift too far from myself again. If you haven't yet discovered that place – it's there.

SAY GOODBYE TO BEING A VICTIM

At some point, I decided I no longer wanted to be a victim. That sounds easy but it was really hard. Being a victim had been a very comfortable place for me, it hadn't got me anywhere though and I needed to re-build my life. I didn't know how and even though being a victim wasn't pleasant, I still had to mourn the loss of it and say goodbye.

Being a victim makes your world very small. It was a negative place, a world without friends, I had no social life at all and a lot of problems with my sisters and mother. And because I didn't know where I wanted to go in life or how to build my life up, I started with finding out what I didn't want anymore.

First of all, I looked for the good in my situation... I was still standing, I still had a job, I still had a place of my own, that was a start...I learned not to be so ungrateful and negative all the time.

I didn't want to fight with my mother all the time anymore and I began to work on that. I tried to see that what she did and said was for my own good and that she loved me.

And really nothing changed overnight but I took it further: I tried to make friends by doing things I'd never done, I went on daytrips with organisations, holidays with groups and I found colleagues I could relate to.

It has been hard but it's so been worth it, it was a gift to myself really.

THERE'S A BIGGER PICTURE

When I was young, I always dreamed of a fairy tale life: a handsome man, a big wedding, a cute house and a bunch of children. The older I got, I still didn't have a serious relationship and my chances were getting smaller and smaller.

By the time I got ill and still didn't have a serious relationship, I felt a bit of a lost cause. By the time I was forty, I said goodbye to my dream of becoming a mother. I still regret that I don't have children of my own but there was a lesson...a regular life was not meant to be for me, I see that now.

I don't think I could have managed a household in that period of my life and I can honestly say now that I am so happy with my life as it is. I have a rich and happy life and I've learned to get to know myself better. I've discovered what makes me happy and I do those things, I travel alone, I walk a lot, I spend time in nature and read so much.

A big part of my happy life has been accepting who I am, including the fact that I'm a high sensitive person. I set boundaries and plan me-time, I don't do things out of duty or because someone expects me to and I make the most out of any given situation.

So, even though you can't see it at the time, there's a big picture, try to see that.

THE RIGHT TIME WILL COME

When I was a teenager, I wanted to study psychology. It was a turbulent time though and my parents advised me against it, they were scared for me, they knew I still had so much to learn in life. Looking back, they were right and I ended up studying economics and languages.

All these years later though and after a lifetime of learning, I'm still drawn to Psychology: the human mind is like a magnet for me, I can't read enough about it.

The big difference now, is that I've grown into a strong woman, someone not easily carried away with another's story. I know now who I am and what I'm worth. The time is right now to study this amazing topic – with experience and level-headedness.

Sometimes the path to what we want, isn't a straight, direct one but in the end, one can't ever deny what's in the blood. The path I took was the right one, it's never too late and you're never too old to do what you wanted all those years ago, you will too when the time is right.

WHEN YOU CHANGE INSIDE YOU, THE WHOLE WORLD AROUND YOU CHANGES TOO

A few years ago, I went on my personal development journey. Through ill health, I'd been in survival mode for at least a decade and I felt my own personal development was stuck at around age twenty-eight.

Through this work, I discovered I had so much anger in my body, I was angry all the time! I'd had several jobs that I'd left feeling angry about, I was sent to a psychologist at one point to help me but honestly, I knew that wasn't what I needed.

A year later, I met a wellness coach and we worked through so many issues that cropped up in every day real life situations...frustration, anger, feeling like my needs weren't being met. Together, we peeled the layers off the proverbial onion and came to the core.

The bottom line was that I had neglected my own opinions, my own needs, my whole life. Looking back, I think my health issues were attributed to not listening to myself and all that anger had built up.

I didn't want to be angry anymore and thank God, I'm not. My family and good friends really stayed with me through those years, I've seen big changes in my life and I have a different way of looking at the world now: instead of seeing problems, I see the beauty of life.

When you change inside, the whole world around you changes too.

YOU'RE THE ONLY ONE WHO REALLY KNOWS YOUR BODY

Twice, I have known something was wrong, that I was ill and I went to see my GP. He didn't hear me, he said there was nothing wrong with me and he didn't take me seriously on either occasion. I persisted though and I was right. I had serious illnesses and eventually, I got the treatment I needed.

When you feel something is wrong, trust that you're the only one who really knows your body. Even if the world around you is telling you that it's in your head or it's not that serious, keep listening to your body and intuition.

This voice inside me was so loud, I couldn't ignore it and I persisted. Trust your body, trust your gut feeling. You know your own body best.

It's never too late

"I hope my words normalise some of the issues that we face as women. I hope it illuminates the path for someone or lightens the load in some way".

Tricia saw the call to gather here as she was turning fifty and wanted to do something special –
her chapter it is.

Guided by Spirit and her earthly teachers to step in and be seen, she has been a voice for so many in her life, not least for her daughter who has a rare disability.

Her husband, Greg, is a constant support to her as they have met and got to know the many different versions of themselves
through the years. Tricia is an inspiration, we hope her words find your heart.

@tricia_allen_therapies

TRICIA ALLEN

SET AN INTENTION AND DARE TO DREAM

For many years I had dreamt of developing groups, where people could come together and embark on personal development. I wanted to combine what I knew about Psychotherapy and Spiritual health and make pleasant experiences where people could learn about themselves and grow.

I would always find reasons to put it off. All kinds of negative thoughts and processes ran through my head but in truth, I was scared of branching out for fear of negative judgement and failure.

I started to notice people's wellbeing decline a few years back and it gave me the push I needed to get started. My first attempt was to offer free Mental Health support groups. These were poorly attended and I knew this was down to the stigma associated with it...in truth, it didn't feel right to me either. Too wooden, too much like what I'd done in past therapeutic roles.

I realised that if I really wanted something different (which I totally did) I'd just have to start, even if it was the tiniest step. I reached out for some Cacaoista training and began further Shamanic Training.

I hold a deep passion for plant medicines, they have been such a powerful therapeutic part of my personal healing journey, I know I had to blend my two passions. Ceremonial Cacao had been a strong teacher plant for me, I personally knew the benefits, so it fully aligned. I put on some local cacao ceremonies and eventually they became a regular thing.

I set the intention and I dared to dream, you can too.

LEARNING TO BE FLEXIBLE AND CHECK IN

Growing up in different environments, it is inevitable I think, that we each develop a unique set of rules for living, that we each find our own way of judging ourselves and others. As we age, I feel like we internalise these rules to the point that they become invisible. I feel it's like trying to see the air we breathe or asking a fish what water is!

I've found that I most often notice my own conditioning when someone upsets me. If someone breaches an expectation of mine or I feel they're failing to measure up in some way.

One of the many personal lessons I've learnt over the years, is that it's not the situation I find myself in that causes distress but my beliefs about it. If I can find a way to change my perspective to something more rational, I often feel better quite quickly.

Revisiting my rules of living, my 'should's', 'musts' and 'ought to's', help prevent me from being too rigid in my thinking. I've learned to check in and be flexible, that might be what you're being called to do right now.

YOUR CHILDREN WILL APPRECIATE EVERYTHING YOU DID WHEN THEY'RE OLDER

Mothering is an art not a science. There are moments when I've felt like I'm doing great and inevitably times when I've struggled to know how to do it. All entirely normal and if you feel like that, you're not on your own.

I think we're all winging it! My days have been spent prepping for my children, doing laundry, shopping, cooking and cleaning. We did the parents evenings, nights out with my husband where we just talked about the kids (rather than immersing yourselves in one another's embrace) and what I've realised is that it's truly impossible, no matter what you do, to please your children all the time.

In fact, I think much of what parents do to ensure their children thrive goes completely unnoticed by them. It won't be until adulthood or even when they become parents, that they might acknowledge what we did. Don't take it personally if your children aren't witnessing your effort or sacrifice. The paradox is, the fact that they can't see it means you're doing a really great job!

They might only be grateful for all the clean clothes, the food on the table and the access to an education and the love they got, once they've grown up. My kids are grown up now and I feel my worth. I know they felt my love and I know that the invisible (to them) offerings are greatly appreciated in adulthood.

TRUST AND SURRENDER IF YOU FEEL CHANGE COMING ON

I made the decision to change career direction. Every fibre in me knew it was the right time to make a change but I worried about how this would impact my finances, my children and my partner. What people would think also concerned me and my job had become part of my identity, it had status with it. I wrestled and struggled with it for some time. But here's the thing, my body was already telling me, I knew!

I just had to leave, ignoring it was making me ill. I know that when my body communicates with me through illness, I just have to tune in, trust and surrender to the change.

LOVE DEEPLY AND ALSO KEEP SPACE TO LOVE YOURSELF FULLY

Over the years, I've come to realise that betrayal and disappointment in relationships are probably inevitable. In my experience, people rarely live up to the expectations of others, how can they? They have their own visions, which don't always align with those around them.

People are constantly evolving and changing, so much so, that life is a continual process of beginnings, middles and endings. I've learned not to struggle so much with the 'what if love goes wrong' thoughts and I concern myself more with 'what resilience do I have to cope, when this love changes or even slides away?'.

I don't believe it's 'love' that hurts, I think love is beautiful, I believe it's the unpredictability of relationships and our need for attachment to another that can be brutal – and the fact that I think humans can really struggle with change and endings.

It's a dance between wanting the warmth of another and keeping our whole Selves as independent, resilient entities.

If these words are ringing true for you, keep your own sovereignty and direction. Keep space to love fully in partnership and also space to love fully by yourself. You are you and I am me, in the middle there is a 'we'.

FIND CONNECTION IN THE MOMENT

I have come to learn, that it's in the stillness of the moment, that I consciously create for myself and that I can be in true alignment. Being in alignment with me, brings me peace and headspace. My world, like yours, can be filled with good, bad, chaos, all kinds of dynamics but in the stillness of the moment, there is peace and an escape from anxiety and depression.

If, however, stillness is hard to find, I bring forth the knowledge of mindlessness. I believe it to be the art of fully capturing the moment, to the point of saturation. Like stillness, it can free us from both the past and the future, it can be a beautiful thing.

The idea is that if you can fully distract or mesmerise yourself with things that interest you, things that make you laugh, things that demand your concentration, you can attain the kind of connection that stillness brings.

Sometimes my mindfulness is painting, sometimes dancing, listening to poetry, drumming, playing guitar, it varies every day. The main thing, is creating the moment and giving yourself some time. Find connection with yourself in the moment, therein lies the treasures of your inner wisdom.

MUSIC IS MEDICINE

It was in a Shamanic ceremony that I got the call. The plant spirit spoke to me, saying 'you need to sing and play guitar'. Instantly I recognised that music was going to be a vehicle for my spiritual channelling. I just didn't know how to sing or play guitar!

I was forty-seven years old, fresh out of Ayahuasca ceremony, in a guitar shop. As I looked about the shop, there was a guitar that kept grabbing my attention. It wasn't on the main display but my eyes kept going back to it. After a bit of deliberation, I bought it and headed home!

I started simply with daily practice. Just persevering, then one day, it started to piece together. I play guitar for me. It's a vehicle for me to connect with my guides and in those moments (where I'm at one with the guitar), I channel my songs.

A lot of songs are just for me, others stick in my ear and I find myself repeating the lyrics over and over again, that's when I know I need to capture the channel.

The songs I create are medicine for me and the listener. My process is, that I sit on the floor and open a sacred space by creating an altar, lighting a candle, burning sage and having my guitar with me.

I set my intention 'to channel music' and I wait. I play, tune in and just allow any words or sounds to flow, there's no 'trying', just flowing. These are the moments where magic happens. Flow is where I find the channel.

LIFE STORMS ARE CYCLICAL AND WILL ALWAYS BE YOUR PUSH TO A DEEPER VERSION OF YOURSELF

There have been times when things have happened suddenly, seemingly coming out of nowhere, hitting me like a destructive storm, there I've been thinking I'm somewhere nice and all of a sudden, the Universe gives me a metaphorical smack around the head!

In some of my most major shit storms, they have honestly felt like the worst things ever... I couldn't see anything in front of me, never mind the next step ahead...like my entire life was slipping through my fingers... I've had no clue what to do.

Some of them were so big, I knew life would never be the same again. Just know this...it's part of time. Just take one day at a time darling. Be your own best friend. Be kind to yourself, be forgiving of yourself. Remember 'nothing stays the same forever' and 'this too shall pass' because it doesn't and they do...these moments are happening for you to grow and experience new things.

Honestly, you'll look back with hindsight and honour this initiation. If you're in the middle of turbulence, just for now, my advice is to go into nature and sit on the earth or under a tree.

Trees help us to see cycles. Spring, Summer, Autumn, or Winter. Sometimes trees teach us that they lose their leaves in order to renourish the Earth. The wisdom comes from knowing the difference between these cycles and matching them onto our situation. In my darkest times I've transformed in ways that I could never have imagined.

The 'no choice' of these situations has been my push. I see now they had to happen so I could transition, learn and adapt.

Without these moments I could never have become this version of myself and this version of myself is awesome.

"True story: I had literally just built my new desk, setting the intention to use it to express myself more fully, when two hours later the invitation to write this book came in. How could I possibly say no?"

Micala's words in this chapter were written at that very desk, flowing directly from her heart to yours. In her work, she advocates for healthier life decisions, with her loudest roar always reserved for her children.

She wishes you an exhale, a release and a breath of fresh air as you read her words, knowing you are seen, you are heard and you are not alone.

@micaladuvoux

MICALA DUVOUX

FIND TRUE KNOWING

I have a voice inside my head that behaves like a back seat driver, trying to grab the steering wheel of my life. The voice is loudest in my most challenging times. It refers me instantly to the wounds that hurt most, for example, 'You see? You are unlovable!'... 'See, you're not safe'.

That back seat driver wants to make my decisions from those stories. It makes me want to act rashly or quieten myself, be nice to prove my worth. But I've realised that making decisions by listening to that voice can be disastrous.

I've seen many people go through their lives acting on the advice of that constant chatter. It really takes awareness to separate the voice chatter from your true knowing.

If you resonate with this, give yourself time and space when making decisions. Write down what the voice is saying, start each sentence with 'the voice says...' and it can help you recognise the story patterns and begin to distance from it.

I believe, our innate guidance system, our true knowing is connected to a higher power and a unique path. While the negative voice is situated in our head, true knowing is centred in our heart. True knowing is calm, sure and rooted in love.

Decision making from true knowing is a whole different frequency. It requires getting still, quiet and going inwards. I like to place my hands over my heart centre and just breathe.

When we stop making so many of our decisions from that hurt and wounded voice, we start the long journey home to ourselves.

YOU ARE INHERENTLY WORTHY OF BEING HERE

One day, I was walking the dogs in the forest behind our home, contemplating worthiness and how out of reach it felt to embody it.

I was drawn to a big pine tree and clarity came: 'Go inwards. Place a loving hand and your attention on your heart. Gently move the brambles of inadequacy and shame to one side. What do you notice?'

I noticed how tall the tree was and how unfurled its branches were, taking up its natural space in the forest. Unworthiness and shame simply didn't exist there. These words are man-made, synthetic concepts made up by humans, keeping us limited, constricted and small. When this lesson was revealed, it was as if worthiness settled in the place where shame had once lived.

Having evolved with nature, I have, we all have, the right to grow tall and unfurl our branches, taking up our natural space. Each of us inherently worthy to be here.

INVITE IN GRACE

It seems to me that none of us have everything together. Such a huge part of our human experience seems to be living with and learning through enormous trials and heartbreak, while trying to get on with daily life.

With working from home and watching social media 'perfectness', I have found it's easy to lose the literal, physical pulse of what real humans are really going through. I often wonder what would happen if we all had more grace for each other as human beings, collectively trying to make our way through, each of us on our own life roller coaster.

One of my favourite places to be is at the arrivals gate at airports. Grace is visible and tangible there, when in the moment the doors slide open and people embrace each other, everything else is forgotten; the journey, grudges, worries, struggles, pain. We simply have grace for each other.

For me, it's so easy to extend grace and compassion to others but turning that in on myself has been a different story. I haven't always been so loving of my own mistakes and yet it's impossible to go through life without failing at something! Failure is where we learn to do differently next time. When I can't access self compassion and grace, I tend to go to those who have my back, no matter what.

They beam love into me, melting my hard edges, giving me courage to move forward. There are people like that in your life too. Lean into them. Be vulnerable (discerningly). If you can't have grace for yourself, let their love wash the mistakes away.

IF NOT NOW, WHEN?

Every year on my birthday, I used to create a list of things I wanted to do before my next birthday. Small things like growing tomatoes and having kitchen dance parties with the kids and bigger experiences, like going on a retreat or learning a new skill.

I would illustrate the list and stick it on the wall, somewhere visible, to keep the seeds alive and I'd tick them off as I went. It created a lot of satisfaction and fun.

I don't know what year I stopped making these lists but it's been a while. Somewhere in the midst of raising my beautiful children, I forgot about my joy while prioritising theirs. Turning fifty however, feels like a new beginning, so I ask myself 'What am I still waiting for?', 'What am I still afraid of?' and 'What stories are still playing that make me want to contain myself, rather than set my whole Self free?'.

I'm creating a new list.

- I want to be in circles of women talking about business
- I want to vagabond (wander around the world) with my husband
- I want all my gifts to be used well, not just for my family but in overflow to others
- I want to create a flower garden
- I want my creative expression and budding faith to lead my way through life
- I want to feel strong and powerful in my body
- I want to hug my friend in the US

"If not now, then when", sings Tracy Chapman. If not now, then when indeed.

FIFTY IS THE BEGINNING OF ADULTHOOD!

I turned fifty this year. While this manmade calendar digit change didn't make a difference to me mentally, I've been noticing some radical shifts in my mind that I'm very much enjoying and wasn't told about.

Before this and despite all the years of personal development, I would still tell myself I wasn't whole. I let other people's perspective of me define me as a person and simultaneously tried to control what people thought of me, by being nice.

I waited for someone, anyone, to give me the permission slip to be truly myself. What I've noticed since turning fifty is that the resistance to step into the wholeness of being me is dissipating. It's getting easier to access self-compassion and acceptance. It turns out the permission slip to be me that I constantly sought outside of myself, was engraved into my cells all along. All it would have taken was my inner knowing of that.

It's as if my DNA was always timed to open and blossom now, at fifty. It feels like I'm just beginning life as a fully fledged adult, anchored into my innate gifts, strengths and life experiences. Fifty isn't so much an accumulation of years but rather an unravelling of the untrue stories I told myself.

Biologically, physically, turning fifty and transitioning into menopause is quite the journey to say the least but it does come with extra gifts that we weren't told about before. Perhaps the next fifty years are all about living and sharing them.

LISTEN TO YOUR BODY

There's an energetic price to pay for not living life true to yourself and I've paid it. A few years back, I found myself pinned to my bed, totally exhausted and in a scary and dark place mentally.

My wise body has always given me signals about what's life giving and soul sucking. The problem was I had been ignoring them and always putting others first. I'd always said yes because I was afraid to say no. I stayed in social groups because I wanted people to like me. My body showed me that my people pleasing and constant proving of my worth had to stop.

I pictured myself flattened out, like a cartoon character that had been run over by a steamroller. I started to pay attention, in my body, to what gave me energy and what drained it. This created an awareness of the things, activities and people that lit me up while others made me exhausted.

I had changes to make. It required taking full ownership of my life force energy. I stepped away from my business, relying on my husband's income and the residual income I had created to live on. I pulled out of groups and gave myself the space my body craved but my mind judged.

Today my life and energy generally feel spacious and peaceful. Even though it was difficult to go through, it was worth listening to the warning signs my body gave me. Is your body giving you signs that something needs to change?

BE YOURSELF AS A PARENT

When my children came along, my inner knowing was solid, I wanted to stay at home to raise them. I was with them all the time and that meant, as they grew up, I saw how they were as true to their unique strengths and gifts as they could possibly be. And as I observed and parented them to stand in that, I also had to stand in my own true self too. It's been SUCH a journey to understanding and accepting myself.

These are the things I learned about myself...

- I'm not a natural nurturer, at least not after my kids were toddlers, it took a lot to accept that about myself. What I did instead was empower them in their next developmental or learning/unfurling phase.

- I'm not frequently sociable. No matter how much I wanted to fit in with the local mums (who met three times a week!), I couldn't! It was exhausting! Instead, I was grateful to have met a mum like me, who made the best cappuccinos and together, we'd sit quietly on her deck, while our kids played.
- I need space...even from the people I love the most...in order for me to recuperate and regenerate. This has been a huge, ongoing, permission slip situation. My family feels the same actually, so they totally accept my need but a part of me still feels bad.

Today, my kids are happy, confident, amazing teenagers. How I've parented them is a huge part of my purpose, legacy and who I am. It's not been secondary to the work I produce but integral.

Society has a lot to say about motherhood. I'm not sure any of us can really win if we listened to everything. All we can do, is navigate parenthood with our unique strengths, gifts and character.

HOW TO GRIEVE A LIVING LOVED ONE

While my higher Self knew the most loving thing to do was to let go of the relationship, that it was the most peaceful way forward for all concerned, it has been brutal for the human, day-to-day part of me.

I've been through the whole range of emotions.

- I miss their sweetness.
- I'm mad at them for never standing up for me.
- I'm grateful for our journey together.
- My heart doesn't understand their lack of grace.
- The silence has been agonising.

Grieving a living loved one has been a very lonely journey. There's shame about how it got to this point. It's reinforced my mind's story of being unlovable and unworthy. As a preventive measure, my heart started to slowly close to other loved ones in my life. However, what I have learned, is that my capacity to give and receive love is not measured on how healthy my relationship with this person is.

That someone cannot love me wholeheartedly, has nothing to do with how good a person I am. As with all grief, I've moved through stages. I'm getting to the acceptance part now, where I accept it's over and I'm keeping my heart open. The silence is less deafening and peace is filling the void.

My focus is shifting towards knowing I am wholeheartedly lovable and worthy, no matter who loves me or not. As are you.

In contributing to this book, Emma
sees herself as a voice for the
women who find life challenging,
for the ones who don't know where
to go or which way to turn.

Throughout her life, whenever she
has witnessed injustice or
unfairness, her internal tiger has
roared into action.

She has consistently stood tall,
never hesitating to defend others,
her voice amplifying with each
passing year.

May her words give you another
perspective, may you feel safe to
think about life differently,
may you feel inspired.

@e.m.m.a.b.o.a.r.d.m.a.n

EMMA BOARDMAN

WORDS ARE MAGIC, CHOOSE THE WORDS YOU SPEAK AND THINK WISELY

I can't remember when it was that I learnt about the magical power of words but I immediately became very conscious about every thought that came into my mind and every word that came out of my mouth.

Have you ever heard someone talking badly about somebody else? To me it feels ugly and low vibration. Not only that but I've wondered what on earth they'd be saying about me when I leave the room!

Then there's the opposite end of the spectrum, the beautiful one who speaks every word with love and kindness, it feels as though they're sending such loving frequencies into the world.

I have a friend who's constantly complaining - about anything and everything - and funnily enough, her life keeps giving her lots of things to complain about. It's as if she invites a constant cycle of negativity into her life.

If we really do have the power to choose the thoughts and words that directly impact and shape our world, then surely we only want to be thinking and saying the loveliest of things, right?

I invite you to carefully consider all the words you think and speak from here on. If you focus on all your words coming from a place of love, I assure you, you'll see the most profoundly positive impact on your life.

DARE TO DREAM REALLY, REALLY BIG!

I didn't see much inspiration around me growing up; it all seemed too simple, too safe and too uninspiring.

Yet in my head; I was dreaming of a life that was off-the-charts, I wanted glamour, excitement and adventure, all the things that were not in my home town of Dorset. I remember being a little girl and dancing around the living room in my pyjamas watching Top of The Pops on TV and imagining that I was one of those fabulous dancing girls.

When I told people what I wanted to do, they laughed at me and told me to get realistic - that made me want it even more. Despite the odds, I managed to secure a place at a top London dance college. I worked really hard over the three years and when I left college, I started the audition process and I DID end up being one of those glamorous girls you see dancing on TV!

Dream after dream became a reality and I soon began to realise the magic of clearly visualising the next steps in life. I did lose my way sometimes, it happens. I found myself in relationships living somebody else's dream but I always got back on track by continuously dreaming and imagining the next chapter and making choices that steered me in their direction.

My own experience has proven that the state of our past or our current situation does not in any way dictate our future. Our dreams are always in our hands and it's up to us to make them a high priority.

So please, never stop dreaming. Always remember to dream your dreams a size too big so you can grow into them. That's where the magic really happens.

SHOULD YOU HAVE A BABY?

There are a few subjects in life that everyone has an opinion on. Having a baby is one of them. Society expects that women of a certain age will have a child, if they're able and most women I knew in my twenties and thirties were aching to have a baby in their arms. I definitely wasn't one of them.

To me it all sounded very inconvenient. I was trying to build a career and have a good time! It wasn't until I was forced to close my company and my boyfriend proposed out of the blue, followed by a whirlwind wedding that left me in a new role as a housewife, that I found myself being asked the question, "Shall we try for a baby?".

For someone who'd never dreamt of pushing a buggy down the street or even once glanced in baby shops, this question was quite tricky. I didn't really, really want one but I didn't really not want one either - I guess you could say I was in neutral territory.

I decided that it was a wonderfully romantic thing to do, so I agreed to try. Becoming a mother was challenging and beautiful in equal measures. It made me a much less selfish person. Being responsible for someone else's life gets you out of your own head like nothing else.

If you're on the fence about having a baby, I share my experience in the hope that if you're in neutral territory, like I was, you'll consider the experience. To witness a life lived from the beginning, brings a new appreciation for the utter magic of life itself.

REFRAME YOUR THINKING, YOUR PARENTS DID THEIR BEST

My parents spent most of my childhood at war with each other. My sister and I got accustomed to sleeping with our heads under the pillow to save ourselves from the sound of doors slamming and constant arguing.

After being caught a few times in the crossfire of flying objects, I learnt it was best to stay out of the way! I tried to tell them their behaviour was upsetting but they were so caught up in their anger and frustration, they were not able to behave any differently.

It was quite a chaotic homelife. My father used to buy run-down properties, transform them, make them beautiful, then sell and repeat. We lived in them during all the reforms, so brick dust and cement always brings childhood memories flooding back.

Life calmed down a bit when they finally divorced when I was eleven, there was less shouting and we lived a more settled life with my mum. In my twenties, an older friend asked me to share about my relationship with my parents. After I told him, he responded in a way that completely shifted my perspective.

He said grown-ups, especially parents, are only ever doing what they can with the awareness they have. He also said that my frustrating and dysfunctional upbringing had served as the dynamo for my life and I should be grateful for the drive it had given me.

His comments opened my heart to a completely new perspective I'd never considered. I felt immediately softer towards them and most of my frustration melted away.

The rest of the forgiveness came when I had my own son. I realised what a minefield parenting actually is and how we're ALL only doing the best we can, with the awareness we have at the time. If you're still angry at your parents for whatever reasons, I invite you to try and reframe your thinking, your parents did their best.

TIME TO SAY NO

I was a total 'yes' girl. I said yes to everything, the projects, the parties, the opportunities and all the stuff in-between. I thought the word 'no' was for losers, that was until I realised, it was the only word that was going to save my life.

Years of hustling, burning the candle, hitting a wall, taking a break when illness struck only to repeat it all, again and again, was a standard part of life. It wasn't until the age of forty-seven, when the burnout of all burnouts finally taught me to unapologetically say the word No!

I woke up in hospital to discover I had dangerously high levels of bacteria in my bloodstream, caused by a sepsis infection on my only kidney. I was stunned how a mild UTI could get so out of control.

My body had been whispering to me to stop but I didn't listen, I was too busy trying to fulfil my business obligations and please the people who'd invested in my company. I'd never had investors in any businesses before and I felt as if they owned me.

It was only when I realised how fragile my life was, that I finally felt the strength to say no to my business obligations.

Sending the email to my investors while on an IV drip in the hospital bed was the biggest thing I'd ever done. Saying no to others while saying yes to myself was a new thing for me, a huge breakthrough and one that has become my new mantra. I am now on a NO mission, I always say NO to the things, people and places where my health, well-being or sanity feels compromised.

Saying NO to the wrong stuff gives us space to say YES to the right stuff. And having space to say YES is so important, it's where we find the opportunities, abundance and magic.

DON'T CHASE THE MATERIAL STUFF

My obsession with wealth started when I was young, fascinated by mums' rich friend who, in contrast to our life of financial struggle, seemed to be living a peaceful life filled with grace, ease and abundance, I couldn't wait to be grown up and live a fancy life!

I was attracted to the cocky swagger of my first serious boyfriend, he was as wealth obsessed as I was and we set out on a wild and crazy adventure. Both London entrepreneurs, addicted to the hustle, crazy nightlife and the drive to achieve, we bought properties, leveraged one mortgage against another and racked up some serious credit card debt.

We got married and I became a mum. One day, I found myself alone with my baby, feeling tearful and helpless in the beautiful garden of our large family home, I wondered why this didn't feel as magical as I'd hoped. My husband was working long days to finance our lifestyle and I felt guilty feeling so unhappy, lonely and uninspired, when from the outside, it looked as though I was living the dream.

I was craving more from life; more meaning, more purpose and more connection to something bigger than all of this, I just didn't know where to start looking.

After a bid to slow things down and reconnect with my husband, we moved to Mallorca but a larger property and two swimming pools later, I felt like I was living a nightmare.

Leaving my marriage was the only way and I've since learned that there are much better ways to feel wealthy and none of them involve money! My home is smaller, life is quieter and my car is older...I'm wealthier than I've ever been.

It's ok to say No to Botox!

I'd popped over to a mum-friend's house to pick up my son from a playdate. She invited me inside, asked if I wanted a drink and without skipping a beat, told me it was time I got Botox!

This happened on the week of my forty-ninth birthday. Up until that point, I'd been feeling pretty good about myself but that knocked me sideways for a couple of days and I found myself spending hours, analysing every line on my face, wondering how offensive I must look to warrant such advice.

Fortunately, my self-belief and inner confidence were at an all-time high. I'm so grateful this comment didn't make me go running off to the Botox clinic and hide the treatment from my partner, as she and her friends had done, instead it left me roaring with defiance that I would make a stand for ageing naturally.

I have never once looked at an older woman and seen anything other than her beauty, wisdom and wonder. Every line tells a story and every crease, the result of an emotion felt or a lesson learnt. To erase these natural etches of expression seems like cheating on yourself and disrespecting this wild and wonderful adventure called life. I have friends who weren't so lucky to have made it this far, so I'm ageing for them too.

Fitting in is over-rated

At school, I felt so un-cool, in my jumble sale clothes sporting a home-cut fringe. Mum had a strict no-make-up rule, so with my pale blonde eyelashes and eyebrows, I felt like I had no face! Being a member of the in-crowd looked so enviable. They all seemed better looking, super stylish, witty, popular and cool...somehow, a few years older than everyone else.

Although I would have loved to have felt prettier and more stylish, I remember thinking their cliquey controlling group behaviour looked quite limiting. I was secretly pleased to be on the outside, making my own choices. Abandoning the quest to be cool, is one of the most wonderful things about getting older, the feeling of needing to fit in has faded away and I'm proud to be the odd one out.

I'm so grateful I never compromised myself to fit in to any cliquey groups, I cherish my individuality and feel it's become one of my most powerful assets in life and business. I have wonderful friends, in all different places, who get me. You'll never find me hanging out with the same five people, in the same place every week, talking about the same kind of stuff.

Don't worry about not fitting in. Believe me, it's a blessing! A sign that you're destined to shine brightly in your own unique way. You'll find your people, just carry on being truly you, there'll be some wonderful people who will love you exactly the way you are.

Using her voice powerfully and decisively, Katharine has demonstrated resilience in numerous pivotal moments. Through her divorce, stepping up to lead a ceremony and speaking publicly about shungite, essential oils and bio-resonance, she uses her voice wisely to educate and inspire.

Her words in this book aim to do the same. Believing that everyone has a unique story waiting to be unveiled, Katharine took this chapter as her opportunity to articulate her own.

As you read her words, she wishes you to feel a sense of belonging to sisterhood, knowing that you are not alone and you are supported by every woman who contributed to this book.

@angel.of.wellness

KATHARINE TACON

BE CONFIDENTIAL

'Confidentiality equals Trust.
Trust equals lasting friendships and repeat clients'

That was the best advice I was ever given when I started my first job. My boyfriend at the time said, "Whatever you do, keep confidential information confidential. If you have to break confidence, only do it up the chain of command, never down". This has been ingrained in me ever since. I'm eternally grateful for these wise words.

I joined a management consultancy company as an office junior and within a year, I was promoted to PA to their Operations Director. Soon after that, I got promoted to HR Manager. I was involved in many senior management meetings and was known for being trustworthy.

I've adopted this advice in all areas of my life, throughout my varied employment, with my children, my family, my friends and more recently as a massage therapist and wellness consultant. Now more than ever, confidentiality is important. I live on a small island and many clients confide in me. It's vital that their information remains private and confidential.

Check in with yourself, are you a gossip? Do you disclose private information? Do you talk about others behind their backs? If you do, make a conscious decision to change. Be a role model and lead by example.

BE REALLY AUTHENTIC

What on earth does that mean? How do you become the authentic you? I believe it's all about matching the inside you, with the outside you. It's when the inside version of yourself (the one in the chrysalis of your soul, that may have been suppressed from emerging), shows on the outside too, transforming you into the beautiful butterfly you truly are.

Maybe you don't feel safe to show your true self for fear of judgement or because you're running negative programmes from the past that are hindering your growth.

Sentences that start with 'I can't...wear/say/do/think', follow with 'says who? Who says you can't?'. Remember you are you and no one else on this entire planet is like you, so be you, let your wings unfold and fly. I've found that eliminating words like 'I must', 'I should' and 'I have to' have helped. If you're doing things you don't want to do, to my mind, you're not being your authentic self, you could be people pleasing.

When you practice the art of 'being you, the authentic you', rather than responding to the needs of others, life begins to change and you will feel empowered. Others are more likely to respect you too.

Set some boundaries and follow the fun. It's helped me stand up and become the person I really am, inside and out. You can do it too!

CHOOSE KINDNESS

It doesn't take much to be kind. You simply make a conscious decision to adopt kind words, thoughts and deeds. Life can be really hard, too hard for some to bear and you never know when you'll meet someone close to the edge.

Being kind, all the time, simply means that maybe, one day, your act of kindness could save a life, give hope or joy to someone who really needs it. Unless we've walked a mile in another person's shoes, we cannot begin to understand them. There's no point in being judgemental, we have no idea what anyone else is dealing with. Everyone is doing the best they can, with what they've got. Let them be.

I found the hardest part, was training myself to think kind thoughts about myself! But I learned that my thoughts create my reality, so I'm careful about what I think.

I've also found that forgiveness often overcomes unkindness. Forgiving myself was a really good start. Once I forgave myself, I was freer from anger, frustration and negative thoughts.

Observe your thoughts, witness the negative and replace with the positive, it trains your brain. Go the extra mile...open a door for a stranger, give money to someone in need, say hello more, thank street cleaners and dustbin men. What we put out, we receive. Since I've adopted a religion of kindness, I see kindness all around me. I notice it, observe it, love it and best of all, it's free and addictive!

BE READY TO FORGIVE

The Hawaiian Ho'oponopono - 'pono' means 'balance' (pronounced Ho-oh-Po-no-Po-no). This is a powerful forgiveness mantra, a favourite of mine, it energetically changes negative situations into positive ones.

I have witnessed and heard miraculous stories when people use these simple four phrases:

I'm sorry

Please forgive me

I love you

Thank you

I use them (in any order) when I'm facing a challenging situation, sensing an 'odd vibe', experiencing a problem or encountering conflict.

Here's an example. I went to a café with a friend and the waiter was in a foul mood. He ignored us, was rude to the other customers and was clearly having a bad day. I was explaining that this situation was perfect to use the Ho'oponopono and decided to show her how it worked in practice.

I started to repeat the mantra in my head whilst watching the waiter and sure enough, within a few minutes he came over, apologised profusely and told us that his staff member hadn't shown up, that he was super stressed and was now on his own. He offered us a free piece of cake and couldn't have been kinder for the rest of our visit. We all have the power to change and shift energy. Why don't you give it a go!

TRANSFORM GRIEF INTO NEW LIFE

When mum died, these were just some of the things that upset me:

- watching other people interacting with their mothers
- seeing Mother's Day cards for sale
- Sundays, anniversaries and festive events
- seeing dad move on and get married
- thoughts about joining mum
- the words 'why me, why my mum?'

If you can relate to any or all of the above, my heart goes out to you. They are very normal reactions. It took me a bit of time to work through them but my outlook has completely changed as I've healed. I've turned the negatives into positives and I now find joy.

- I'm grateful to have known my mother, she loved and supported me unconditionally
- I buy Mother's Day cards and send them to mothers I know in need of emotional support or love

- I have my own family now and often invite others who are single or struggling to join us on Sundays
- If I remember, I light a candle and send love on anniversaries and for festive events, I join in and celebrate them
- I'm happy for him that he found love again after such loss and sadness
- She wouldn't have wanted me to join her; she lives on in me
- 'Why me, why my mum?', I now say 'Why not!'. Her death has shaped me to be the person I am today and I wouldn't be living where I am or doing what I do, if she hadn't died.

You see, nothing stays the same. The pain and sorrow won't last forever. Over time, you will heal and find peace. You never forget but you come to terms with their death, you learn and you grow. I certainly did and I will be forever grateful to the best mum ever!

LIFE IS JUST A GAME

Our greatest teachers are normally those closest to us and they're the ones who challenge or trigger us most. If we were to play a game, let's call it 'Your Life' and your soul family decided to play it with you, they'd each choose a role or character to play in your game. They'd take on the role(s) as your mother, father, sisters, brothers, teachers, friends, pets etc.

Next, let's say you had to choose the level you wanted to play - easy, intermediate or advanced - and then what you wanted to experience; love, heartache, travel, sport, abuse, fame etc. Once all this has been agreed, the game begins. The only thing is, you can't recognise your soul family playing their roles as they're all disguised in human form. Throughout the game, you meet them all, playing their roles brilliantly, giving you the experiences you asked for (good or bad). You're learning the valuable life lessons you wanted, growing spiritually, feeling a special connection to someone, as if somehow, you've met them before. The game continues until you die. Imagine then, that when you die, you reunite with your soul family to reflect on what you learnt throughout the game. You can then choose if you want to play again, with a different set of parameters.

I sometimes think of my life like this, it gives me meaning to some of the trials and tribulations I've experienced. It helps me process this thing called 'life' and gives me faith that maybe, just maybe, I'll be reunited with all my loved ones again.

LISTEN TO THE SUBTLE SIGNS

Dying, for the short time I did, was the most incredible, memorable, life-changing experience ever!

It was a lesson and a gift. I was busy at the time. I was everything to everyone, capable but overstretched. I knew I needed to stop, my marriage was a mess and I was exhausted.

I heard my inner voice nudging me to slow down but I didn't react fast enough. Normally when I need to slow down, the Universe will give me a gentle reminder, a sprained ankle or a cut on the hand. This time was different.

I never made it to my last client of the year. I opened our stiff 300 kilo wrought iron gate with vigour but as I turned and walked away, the gate fell, crushing me underneath it. I was knocked out unable to breathe. When I came round, I could see the gate on top of me and realised the situation was serious. The lesson was loud and clear 'Stop!'.

As they operated on my broken body, I was awake. But all of a sudden, the medics stopped and everything went quiet and light, visually and physically, I was totally calm. A wave of peace and love engulfed me and I remember saying "But what about Izzy?", (my nine-year-old daughter). A voice came back, "She'll be ok, don't worry" and I peacefully replied "ok".

I knew I was dying but a crystal ball reader told me I'd live until my 90s! With that thought, a force pushed me backwards and a heaviness returned. Shape, form and dark colours appeared. The next thing I remember, was being back in theatre, singing Christmas carols out loud.

My recovery was challenging but miraculous. Unable to do anything and dependant on my family, I had time to re-evaluate everything, especially my relationship with my husband. We resolved our differences and are now closer than ever. Don't wait for a gate to 'stop' you. Listen to your subtle body and take action.

IT'S OK TO PRESS THE 'FUCK IT!' BUTTON

I've pressed this button a thousand times! It's a mental button I press when I've managed to stop smoking, drinking, overeating, swearing etc and then all of sudden, with absolutely no warning and from deep in my subconscious abyss, a persuasive little devil emerges and I say 'Fuck it!'.

The angel on my shoulder runs and hides and leaves me to face the devil solo. In a trance like state, my self-control vanishes and I hear the words 'Fuck It' and just like that...I'm back to my old unhealthy habits again. This mental battle has been an internal war of mine for years. The self-loathing, disappointment and shame that comes with another failure, used to eat me up for days.

Now, however, rather than beating myself up like I used to do, I simply acknowledge that the devil won this round but, on the whole, more times than not, I win! On that basis alone, I stop dwelling on it and choose to forgive myself. I soon snap out of my negative thoughts and sure enough, my competitive spirit returns to try and try again.

Our last word goes to...

SANDRA CLENNELL

for our final words of wisdom, we come out of Sacred Eldership order,
to give the last words to 'the girl with no voice'

Throughout my childhood I was known as 'the girl with no voice'. An incredibly shy child, my birth father left the scene long before I was born. This was the sixties, my mum was a young single woman and we lived with my grandparents who I adored. She remarried and her new husband scared me a little. He was never an easy man to live with, he had a cutting humour and not an ounce of empathy towards me. I remember my mum telling me she hated precocious children and my best friend died when we were six, as a result of a riding accident, so with all of that, my world was lonely. Fear of abandonment, failure and humiliation lead me to acquiesce and not speaking out became my coping strategy.

It wasn't until in my thirties, that I felt a compelling urge to break my silence. I was in a workshop at work, we were split into teams to each do a project. Someone from each group was to feed back to the whole group at the end.

I was suddenly overcome by this incredible need to be the person who gave the feedback. When it came to our group, I just did it! I spoke for everyone. It was one of THE most empowering moments of my life. I couldn't have stopped myself if I tried, I was on a mission. I found my voice!

So, my words of wisdom for you, the woman who chose so kindly to open this beautiful book at my page, is to 'just do it'! Be yourself. Say what you want to say. Say it kindly but be assertive.

You know...someone somewhere is always going to disagree with you...but someone somewhere is always going to agree with you too. I found out there was no real need to live in fear of speaking up, of saying what I preferred, of asking, of going first or of being the spokesperson. So do it, speak your truth!

I would have loved to have read that when I was younger. I needed permission to use my voice and if you do, consider this your permission.

As a mother, I taught my sons that everyone's perception of reality is their own. If someone disagrees with you, it really is nothing more than their opinion from where they see the world. Others have a different perception than you; they've had a different upbringing, they have a different life lens, they'll naturally see things differently. Disagreements are simply a reflection of their viewpoint, not a personal attack on yours.

I was brought up in a time where women were expected to be agreeable, nice girls. You, dear reader, don't have to be like that. Have fun, enjoy your life, feel successful at being yourself...whether you're an artist or a scientist or a mum bringing up her children, just please your Self.

I firmly believe that our life purpose is to be happy, to actually please ourselves, in peace and in power. I believe that the gifts we were born with, are our reason for being here and learning to feel comfortable in our own skin...that's the journey.

So...be gentle and kind with yourself, use your beautiful voice and please...please your Self.

With my love, Sandra.

...use your beautiful voice

Sincere thanks go to...

EVERY WOMAN INVOLVED
IN THIS BEAUTIFUL BOOK...

Kim Farr founder of Bali Street Mums, Deborah Darling our Spokeswoman and writer of our Foreword, Sandra Clennell who had the last word, Azizi Birkeland for her support in marketing and our photographers: Belinda Grant, Francois Pistorius and Livvie Spall. And of course, our beautiful authors in Sacred Eldership order;

Kate Peace

Sallie Warman-Watts

Philomena Jordan-Patrikios

Elene Marsden

Gudren Otten

Kate 'fluff' Thorne

Annie Slowgrove-Scott

Morna Milton-Webber

Kath Morgan-Thompson,

Mikel Ann Hall,

Karen Pullan

Janine Vine

Jenn Levers

Joy Webb

Prem Devi

Farideh Diehl

Cathy McPherson

Jackie Clifford

Toni Eastwood OBE MBA

Andrea Jackson

Lesley Markey

Mairi Taylor

Jan Calvert

Stevie Foster

Suzy Walker

Tamsyn Stanton

Alena Hawk

Deborah Thomas-Hladecek

Sumi Chatterjee

Rev Deb Connor Li Xiao Yi 笑意

Kerry Walton

Elisabeth de Charon de Saint Germain

Iona Russell

Sue Royle

Carol O'Connor

Lisa Harris

Tara Paonessa

Gus Grima

Martje Manthee

Tracey Vaughan

Elaine Hill

Andrea Fáfnis Ólafs

Alexandra Fraser-Duran

Marjolein Ruiter

Tricia Allen

Micala Duvoux

Emma Boardman

Katharine Tacon

OTHER BOOKS AVAILABLE ON AMAZON ARE:

A Woman's Blessing - Nourishment for the rise of the feminine, by Lynette Allen
HELD - Guidance for the rise of the feminine, by Lynette Allen
Sacred - Integration for the rise of the feminine, by Lynette Allen
The Women who Gathered (book collaboration), curated & edited by Lynette Allen

For more information on Gather the Women sister circles visit www.gatherthewomen.co.uk

And if you would like to be considered for Lynette's next book collaboration project, register your interest via www.awomansblessing.com/bookcollab

Printed in Great Britain
by Amazon